MOTORMASTER

**Pat Langley–Price
and Philip Ouvry**

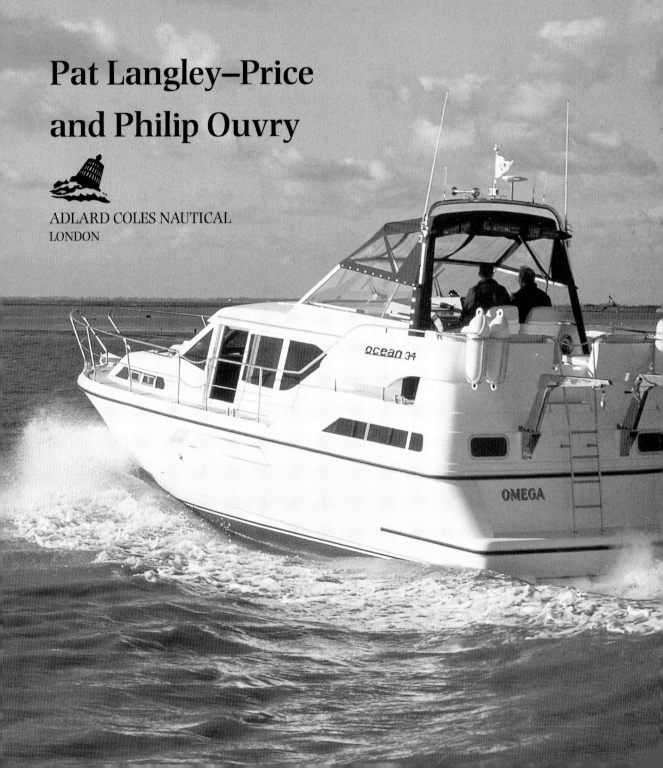

ADLARD COLES NAUTICAL
LONDON

Published by Adlard Coles Nautical 1997
an imprint of A & C Black (Publishers) Ltd
35 Bedford Row, London WC1R 4JH

First published 1997
ISBN 0–7136–4009–X

A CIP catalogue record for this book is
available from the British Library.

Typeset in Photina 10/13pt by Penny Mills
and Falcon Oast Graphic Art
Printed in Great Britain by Butler and Tanner
Ltd, Frome and London

MOTORMASTER

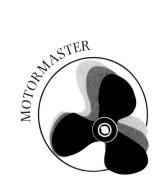

CONTENTS

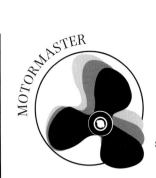

INTRODUCTION

You have often dreamed of transporting your family and friends on relaxing cruises to beautiful scenic harbours and anchorages in your own elegant, gleaming boat. The day has come when you cautiously nose your newly acquired motorboat out of the marina or harbour – your excitement tinged with apprehension. Still, with an experienced, knowledgeable friend or instructor by your side, you will soon gain confidence and get the hang of handling your boat and controlling her engines.

But that is not all you need to know. To ensure that you really enjoy your new boating interest safely you will need to understand the basic navigational concepts and elements of seamanship. This book aims to give you the theory behind these skills.

So, having practised in local waters, you are now ready to venture on your first short voyage. How do you start to plan?

First of all, you will need the nautical equivalents of maps and guide books. Visit your nearest chandlery and you should find racks of marine charts and guide books called pilots, which are the marine versions of route maps and gazeteers. Choose the charts and pilots for the areas where your boat is moored and where you are interested in cruising. When you take them home and study them, a whole new world will start to open up. Even on stretches of coast that you know quite well you will find features that you were unaware of. In the pilot you will find interesting photographs and diagrams plus pages of information about tides, harbour entry signals, approaches, anchorages, berthing and so on.

The principles of seamanship and safe navigation are the same for all vessels whether they are supertankers, motorboats, sailing boats or dinghies. However, the way you navigate will depend on the type of craft you have. The skipper of a 10 metre sailing boat with an auxiliary engine will primarily be concerned with the strength and direction of the wind. As he or she will not expect to achieve speeds of over five or six knots (nautical miles per hour); he will also need to be very aware of tidal streams and currents which will very much affect the boat's speed and direction. On the other hand, a motorboat skipper will be less concerned about the wind because he can motor easily in any direction and his engines can allow him to largely ignore the tidal stream.

One factor that you have to consider is whether there is enough depth of water to allow you to motor where you want to go at all states of the tide. Will your boat be high and dry on a particular mooring and are there any dangerous underwater hazards that you have to avoid? This is where the ability to read the chart for the area is a very important part of your planning.

Are there Rules of the Road at sea? Yes. There is a very well-established set of regulations for preventing collisions at sea and you will need to know these when you come into contact with other vessels. And what of way-finding? On land we have road signs and landmarks but how do we find our way at sea? There is an internationally recognised system of buoyage which helps us to find our way around coasts and into harbours by a visual navigation known as pilotage; there are also seamarks such as beacons and lighthouses to assist us.

Before setting off on a voyage, also known as a passage in nautical terms, good planning is essential, especially when navigating at high speed in a small craft. In a vessel travelling at less than 10 knots it is easy to work out your boat's position, and the direction (course) to steer to reach your destination. Positions are usually worked out on a chart using geographical co-ordinates known as latitude and longitude. Once plotted, these co-ordinates are recorded in a notebook known as the deck log or log book. In a motorboat capable of speeds of more than 30 knots, the distance travelled in the time it takes to work out the boat's present position and course-to-steer can be significant, unless the boat slows down or stops. At higher speeds, therefore, it makes sense to record relative positions such as the distance and direction of the destination or a key position on the way which is known as a waypoint. Modern electronic aids have revolutionised navigation at high speeds though we do stress that it is still important to understand the principles of conventional chart navigation as a back-up in case of equipment failure.

The route you will take is called a passage plan (see Chapter 25 for how to prepare this), and advice on navigating at speeds above 10 knots will be found in Chapter 15.

There is also the subject of weather which, even to a motorboater, is of great importance for the well-being of skipper, crew and vessel. You will probably find yourself taking much more interest in the radio and television forecasts, learning to translate the verbal shorthand of the shipping forecast and constantly looking for weather signs and better and more accurate weather predictions.

Finally, after you have gained knowledge on boat handling, navigation and chart-work, passage planning, tides, collision regulations, pilotage and weather, you will need to ensure that you and your crew are safely equipped to go to sea with the right clothing, adequate fuel, safety equipment, engine spares (and an idea of what to do with them!) first aid supplies and a radio – with current licence for both boat and operator – to summon help in an emergency. This may seem a great deal to learn for a holiday down the coast with the family but as you read through this book and the subjects unfold you will find yourself being drawn into the fascinating nautical world and will be keen to find out more and improve your seamanship.

ROYAL YACHTING ASSOCIATION

For the United Kingdom waters the Department of Transport (DTp) has granted the Royal Yachting Association (RYA) the authority to set the appropriate standards for seamanship and navigation for users of leisure craft. The Royal Yachting Association's Certificates of Comptency, though not mandatory, are internationally accepted as evidence that the holder has the necessary knowledge and ability to carry out safely all the functions set at the appropriate grade. The grades for both sail and motor driven craft are: Competent Crew; Day Skipper; Coastal Skipper; Yachtmaster Offshore; Professional Yachtmaster; and Yachtmaster Ocean. The objective of this book is to give the reader both sufficient information and sufficient exercises to reach the level of theoretical knowledge required for Coastal Skipper/Yachtmaster Offshore Certificate. It also includes the relevant information for the Day Skipper theory certificate. A good skipper or captain of any boat must be aware of many things including the limitations of any other vessels he might encounter. The principles of good navigation and good seamanship are the same for all seafarers no matter what type of vessel they are aboard.

Local or day cruising

The Royal Yachting Association have defined the grade Day Skipper for the seafarer who wishes to skipper a leisure craft in daylight within sight of land. Whilst being aware of the correct actions to take if the weather deteriorates or if overtaken by nightfall, the Day Skipper should be able to find shelter before such events occur.

Coastal cruising

The Coastal Skipper grade is for the more enterprising skipper who will make occasional night passages and short passages out of sight of land, such as a Channel crossing. He will be able to navigate in adverse weather conditions and use all modern navigational aids.

Cruising Offshore

The Yachtmaster Offshore grade is for the more experienced skipper who has extended his cruising horizons to include long passages, maybe remaining at sea for two to three days. It is the qualification which, for a yachtsman, is equivalent to a Master's Certificate in the Merchant Navy.

The Professional Yachtmaster grade is for any Yachtmaster Offshore who wishes to use his qualifications for commercial purposes. He will need the following additional certificates: Medical fitness; Sea survival; Ship Captain's medical course (ocean passages only).

Ocean Passage Making

Yachtmaster Ocean is an extra grade for the skipper intending to make long ocean passages where the principal method of navigation is by observation of celestial bodies.

International Certificate of Competence (ICC)

No certificate of competence is required in the United Kingdom to use a pleasure yacht under 80 gross registered tons. United Kingdom citizens visiting foreign countries may be asked by marine officers for a certificate to show that they are competent to use a boat. The Royal Yachting Association issues the International Certificate of Competence to British citizens to simplify visits to foreign countries. The basis for issuing such certificates is that the applicant can show evidence that he or she is competent to handle the boat under power in confined waters and has a knowledge of the International Regulations for Preventing Collisions at Sea.

KNOW YOUR BOAT

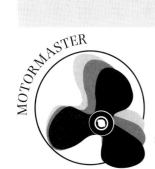

C H A P T E R   O N E

HULL TYPES

Your choice of hull type will depend on what type of cruising you wish to do. Hull design broadly falls into three categories:

Displacement hulls

These operate at speeds up to about 10 knots (nautical miles per hour) and displace their own weight in water with the water parting at the bow and closing in at the stern. As the water is pushed aside waves are created along the length of the hull. As the boat increases speed, these waves also increase until the boat reaches her maximum displacement speed. The boat's maximum speed is closely related to the waterline length of her hull. A boat of waterline length of 25 ft will have a top speed of about 7 knots whereas a 36 ft displacement hull would have a maximum speed of approximately 8.4 knots.

You can work this out using a simple equation: maximum speed in knots equals the square root of the waterline length in feet multiplied by 1.4.

You can see that boats with displacement hulls are relatively slow, so what is their advantage? The main plus point is that they do not require very powerful engines to reach cruising speeds, so that they are economical to run. Another advantage is that they have a fairly deep draft which makes them stable and seaworthy in bad weather.

If you are considering doing most or all of your cruising on inland waters, a boat with a displacement hull is ideal as all waterways have low speed limits to avoid river or canal bank damage or disruption to liveaboard craft. And when cruising down a river why hurry? Relax, just amble along and enjoy yourselves!

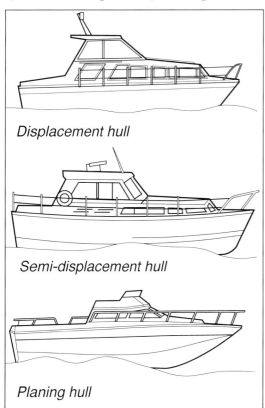

Displacement hull

Semi-displacement hull

Planing hull

Fig 1.1 *Hull types.*

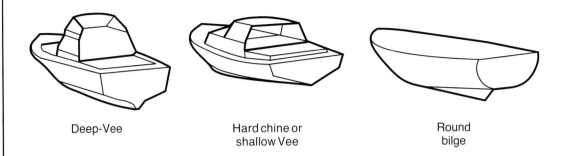

Deep-Vee   Hard chine or   Round
                  shallow Vee   bilge

Fig. 1.2 *Hull shapes*

Semi–displacement hulls

Basically these are heavier craft which travel through the water like the displacement craft but they are designed with a flare to the bow and powerful engines so that part of the hull can lift up out of the water at speed. A displacement hull may be designed with a deep-V bow but a round bilge hull from amidships to stern.

This style of hull is obviously very versatile. It handles well at low speeds on inland waters but punches through waves out at sea.

Planing hulls

Unlike the displacement hull which is constrained by its waterline length, shape and engine power, the planing hull is designed for speed and manoeuvrability. Planing hulls generate vertical lift when the boat reaches its planing speed – lifting the boat out of the water. Once on the plane, resistance from the waves is minimal so that the boat can move even faster over the waves. The ideal planing boat would have a completely flat bottom but would be hard to steer and the occupants would have a very rough ride due to the boat continually slamming. The deep-V hull was designed to maximise speed but also to provide a smoother ride.

This is the type of hull to choose if you would like a smaller boat to go day cruising around the coast or to water ski, or want a larger boat for offshore cruising and entertaining. The disadvantage of the planing-hulled boat is a big thirsty engine!

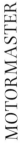

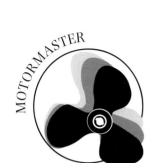

CHAPTER TWO

NAUTICAL TERMS

Areas of the boat

Forward (pronounced for'ard) is the front part of the boat: eg 'I'm going for'ard'.
Bow is the foremost point of the boat.
Aft is the back part of the boat.
Stern is the extreme back end of the boat.
Transom is the flat area across the back of the hull.

Movement and direction

Ahead A term used when the boat is travelling forward ie 'full ahead' – full throttle forwards. It can also refer to an object sighted in a direct line in front of the boat.
Astern refers to the boat travelling backwards or in the direction of an object behind the boat.
Port is the left side of the boat.
Starboard is the right side of the boat.
Port bow is to the left side the bow.
Starboard bow is the right of the bow.
Beam is the width of the boat so 'on the port beam' would be on the left side and 'on the starboard beam' would be on the right.

Hull terms and measurements

Hull describes the body of the boat below deck level.
Keel is the central 'back bone' through the hull.
Stem is the continuation of the keel up to the bow.

Length overall (LOA) is the extreme length of the boat from the foremost part of the bow to the aftermost part of the stern including any projection such as a bathing platform.
Hull length is the length of the hull only, without any projections.
Waterline length or **load waterline (LWL)** is the length of the hull from stem to stern at water level.
Beam overall is the width at the widest outside part of the boat.
Draught or **draft** is the distance from the waterline to the lowest part of the keel.
Displacement The weight of water displaced by the boat which is, in effect, the weight of the boat.
Topsides The sides of the hull above the waterline.
Chine An angle where the bottom of the hull meets the side.
Spray rails Extra angles on some hulls are designed to deflect spray downwards.
Gunwale (pronounced gunnel) is the upper edge of the side of the boat.
Rubbing strake A line of raised moulding, rubber strip or rope along the hull to help protect the topsides from contact damage.
Fenders Any kind of 'buffer' hung along the outside of the hull to prevent contact with piers, jetties and other boats.

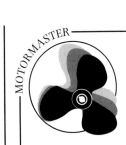

PARTS OF A BOAT

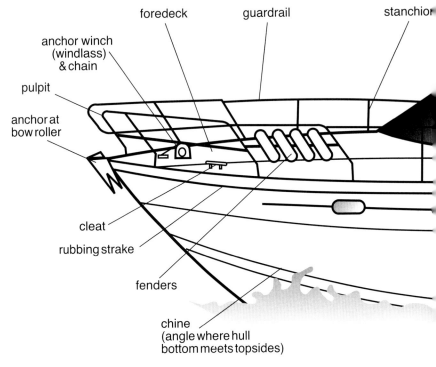

foredeck guardrail stanchion

anchor winch
(windlass)
& chain

pulpit

anchor at
bow roller

cleat

rubbing strake

fenders

chine
(angle where hull
bottom meets topsides)

Now that you are a boatowner you will want to know all about your boat and familarise yourself with all the nautical terms which describe its parts. Here is a sketch based on a Princess 35, a popular cruising boat with a deep-V hull. Turn to the Glossary at the back of the book for more nautical terms.

Above decks

Helm the wheel and steering gear (the tiller in small boats).
Cockpit An open space, below deck level, where the crew can stand or sit and usually contains the helm.
Wheelhouse A weather-proof structure housing the wheel and instruments.
Flying bridge An open steering position, often with a passenger seating area, situated above the wheelhouse.

Coachroof Raised decking above the forward cabin.
Pulpit A frame, usually made from stainless steel, fixed at the point of the bow.
Guardrails Safety lines attached to the pulpit which pass through the eyes of stanchions bolted to the deck.
Gantry A sturdy frame sometimes attached to a flying bridge to house radar, aerials and navigation lights.
Davits A small crane fitted at the stern for hoisting a dinghy.

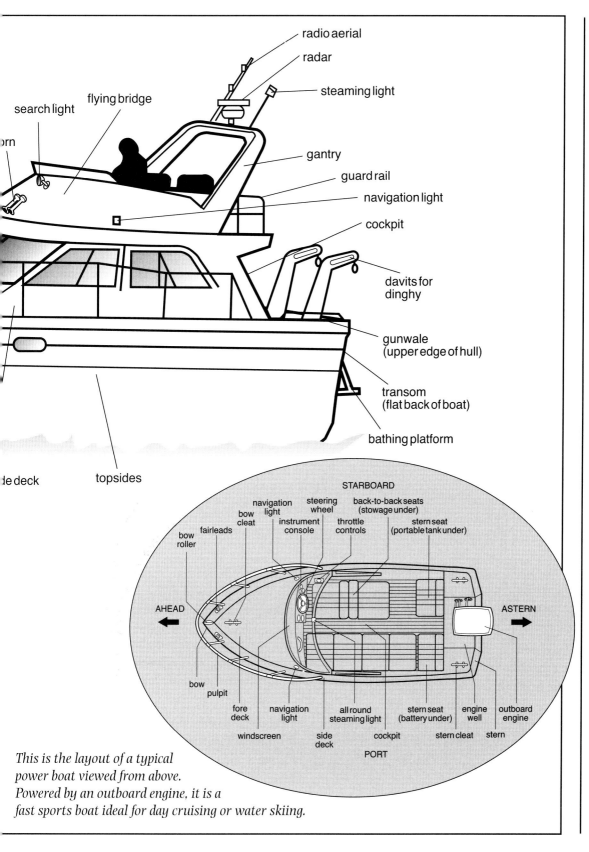

radio aerial

radar

steaming light

flying bridge

search light

gantry

guard rail

navigation light

cockpit

davits for
dinghy

gunwale
(upper edge of hull)

transom
(flat back of boat)

bathing platform

...de deck   topsides

STARBOARD

navigation
light

steering
wheel

back-to-back seats
(stowage under)

bow
cleat

instrument
console

throttle
controls

stern seat
(portable tank under)

fairleads

bow
roller

AHEAD

ASTERN

bow
pulpit

fore
deck

navigation
light

all round
steaming light

stern seat
(battery under)

engine
well

outboard
engine

windscreen

side
deck

cockpit

stern cleat

stern

PORT

This is the layout of a typical
power boat viewed from above.
Powered by an outboard engine, it is a
fast sports boat ideal for day cruising or water skiing.

MOTORMASTER

5

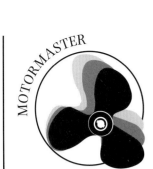

ENGINE CONTROL AND FUEL MANAGEMENT

ENGINE TYPES

Diesel engines

Diesel engines are generally fitted on medium to large displacement and semi–displacement craft. Their main advantage is that they are reliable and economical. Out at sea they are less affected by damp or water penetration than a petrol engine with electronic ignition. Diesel fuel is less flammable than petrol and constitutes less of a fire hazard. Their main disadvantage is that they are heavy and have a slower throttle response than their petrol equivalent.

Four-stroke petrol engines

Petrol engines are generally used for faster, more powerful craft. They are lighter in weight than diesels. Their good power to weight ratio gives good performance and they have a quick throttle response. Their disadvantage is the higher cost of fuel and greater fuel consumption.

Two-stroke petrol engines

Most outboard engines are two stroke, run on a mixture of petrol and oil; the mixture varies between 10:1 (10 parts petrol to 1 part oil) and 100:1. They are comparatively light in weight and the modern engines are very reliable and simple to maintain. They are not fuel efficient so they are relatively expensive to run.

ENGINE CONTROL

A boat's behaviour under power depends on how well boat and engine are attuned. Manoeuvrability is greatly affected by the propeller: a large propeller rotating slowly makes handling easier. Whatever type of engine you have, important points to bear in mind are:

- Carry out regular maintenance, paying particular attention to the prevention of corrosion. Boat engines rarely break down as a result of being used.

- Never run the engine at full speed before it has warmed up; for at least five minutes but ideally 15 minutes.

- Only use 95% of engine speed which is equivalent to 80% of power output; this reserves the 5% for exceptional circumstances. Thermal stresses at maximum speed are very high.

- Carry out regular checks to increase the reliability and durability of the engine. Overloading, caused for example by the fouling of a propeller by seaweed, should be immediately evident and rapid action taken.

If a boat is to be left unattended, then the engine should be run under load for at least an hour at intervals of two weeks and the fuel tanks should be left full. It takes about 14 days for the oil film on an engine to break down allowing corrosion to commence. Any water which has condensed in the sump will boil off after an hour's running. Less condensation will occur in a full fuel tank.

The performance of a power boat depends on a variety of factors: weight, hull shape, smoothness of the hull, propeller design and transmission system. Fig 3.1 shows the interrelationship between boat speed in knots (V), waterline length in feet (LWL), engine brake horsepower (BHP) and displacement in tons (D). The maximum V/√(LWL) ratio will be 1.5 for a displacement hull and 4.0 for a semi-displacement hull.

You can use a simple calculation to work out what size engine your boat will need:

Example: What size engines should be fitted in a 36 ft semi-displacement Customs launch with a displacement tonnage of 20 tons which is expected to have a maximum speed of 24 knots?

Max boat speed/√(waterline length) =

$$\frac{24}{\sqrt{36}} = \frac{24}{6} = 4$$

From Fig 3.1 engine horsepower/displacement = 25

Engine horsepower = $25 \times 20 = 500$

We would expect, therefore, to fit twin 250 bhp engines.

FUEL CONSUMPTION

The more powerful the craft the higher the fuel consumption. Some craft use a gallon of fuel for each nautical mile travelled. In a small craft the performance can be affected significantly by the weight of fuel carried: indeed it may be considered economical to have only sufficient fuel, plus a reserve, for

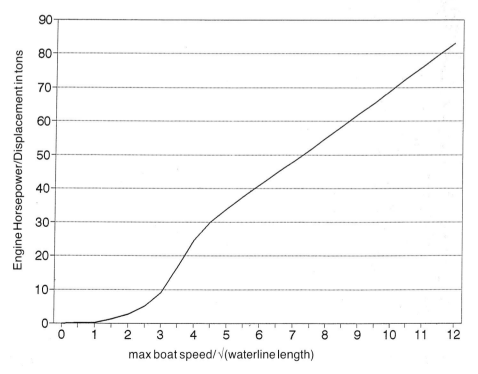

Fig 3.1 *Performance of boat/engine Combinations*

the passage rather than to top up the tanks at the start of every journey. Fuel consumption figures should be available together with an accurate method of measuring the fuel remaining.

All but the shortest passages should include a contingency plan in case of unforeseen events, such as bad weather setting in or the intended harbour being inaccessible, and the amount of fuel carried should allow for any such plan.

Full-speed consumption

As a basic rule of thumb to estimate full-speed fuel consumption, a diesel engine, married to the right propeller and running flat out, will burn about 0.2 litres of fuel per hour per horsepower. Under the same conditions, a petrol engine uses about 0.4 litres per hour per horsepower, and a two-stroke about 0.5 litres per hour per horsepower.

Cruising speed consumption

To work out the economical cruising speed, on a calm day conduct a speed trial to make a table of the engine revolutions per minute (rpm) against boat speed in knots. Figs 3.2 and 3.3 show, plotted as a graph,

typical tables for a planing and semi-displacement (or semi-planing) craft. If the boat speed/engine rpm is plotted against engine rpm, curves are produced (see Figs 3.4 and 3.5) which indicate the most and least efficient engine rpm. From these curves for the planing craft the best performance is at 3900 rpm, which is at 95% full power, and the least efficient engine rpm is around 1700 rpm which corresponds to the speed at which the boat is getting up to the plane. For the semi–planing craft there are two maxima: at 3900 rpm representing the planing mode and around 1500 rpm representing the displacement mode.

The engine performance data given by the engine manufacturer combined with the speed trial results can be used to determine the fuel consumption (litres/hour) and the range (nautical miles per litre). Any theoretical calculations should be checked out in practice by keeping a careful log of the fuel consumed on all major passages.

Volvo Penta have produced a series of curves to calculate the fuel consumption at partial speeds, Fig 3.6. These curves are used in conjunction with the formula:

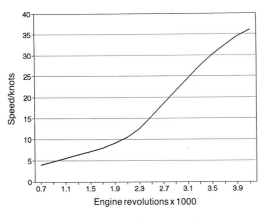

Fig 3.2 *Planing craft.*

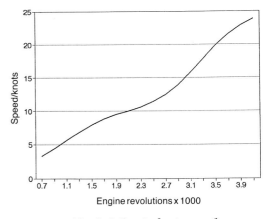

Fig 3.3 *Semi-planing craft.*

MOTORMASTER

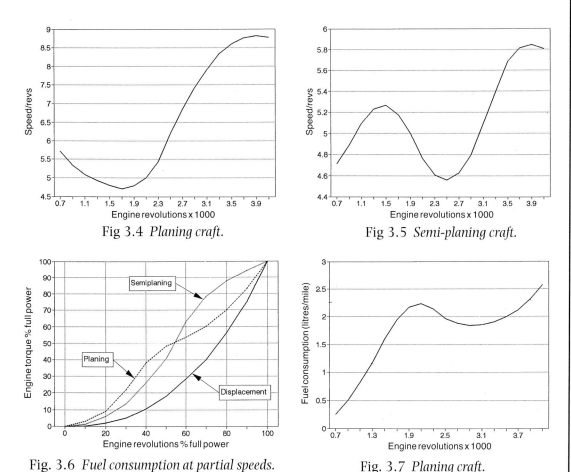

Fig 3.4 *Planing craft.*

Fig 3.5 *Semi-planing craft.*

Fig. 3.6 *Fuel consumption at partial speeds.*

Fig. 3.7 *Planing craft.*

$$\text{Fuel consumption (litres/hour)} = \frac{N_e \times N_2 \times T_2 \times Z}{N_1 \times T_1 \times 830}$$

where: N_e = Engine maximum output (flywheel horsepower)
N_1 = Engine maximum rpm
N_2 = Engine rpm required
T_1 = Engine maximum torque
T_2 = Engine torque at N_2 rpm (from Fig 3.6)
Z = Fuel consumption in *grams/horsepower hour* at engine maximum rpm

Note: N_e, N_1, T_1 and Z are obtained from the engine performance data supplied with the boat by the manufacturer.

By applying this formula to the curves in Figs 3.4 and 3.5, curves of fuel consumption in litres/mile are obtained for planing and semi-planing craft, Figs 3.7 and 3.8. For the planing craft there would appear (Fig 3.7) to be an economical cruising speed at around 3000 rpm (23 knots). For a semi-planing craft the fuel consumption (Fig 3.8) is fairly constant between 3000 and 3700 rpm (14 to 21 knots).

By applying these figures to the fuel tank capacity, operational range can be determined. In practice add a 10% contingency allowance and assume 80% of total fuel capacity is accessible. For the planing craft, Fig 3.9, the economical cruising speed is around 3000 rpm; though, in dire emergency, the range increases significantly below 1500 rpm (7 knots). For the semi-planing craft, Fig 3.10, there is no ideal cruising speed once in planing mode.

Here is an example of a calculation to find out the cruising range for a planing craft fitted with twin 300 litre fuel tanks. You plan to keep a 25% fuel reserve. From Fig 3.7 you can see that the most economical cruising speed appears to be at 3000 rpm where the consumption is 1.8 litres per mile. Your maximum fuel contents would be 600 litres less 25% for your reserve, giving 450 litres available. The cruising range would be 450 divided by 1.8 giving a cruising range of 250 miles. Fig 3.2 gives an equivalent cruising speed of 23 knots.

These curves can be further adapted, if required, to show the maximum economical cruising range for fuel remaining. Such curves give the navigator essential planning information particularly in the situation where it is necessary to know the moment at which the decision has to be made to proceed to an alternative destination.

Note that in a planing boat the weight of fuel carried can make a significant difference to the performance. On occasions it might be sensible only to commence a passage with a partial fuel load; allowing for the increase in performance as the fuel load decreases. If the seas are rough, fuel aeration may well occur as the fuel tanks

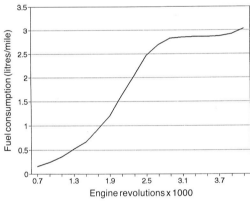

Fig 3.8 *Semi-planing craft.*

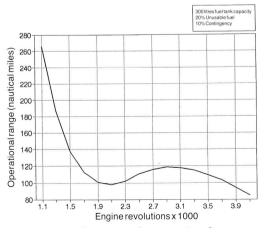

Fig 3.9 *Planing craft: operational range.*

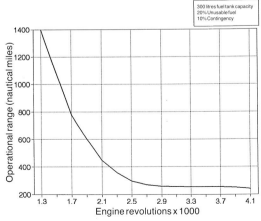

Fig. 3.10 *Semi-planing craft: operational range.*

ENGINE PERFORMANCE DATA

Engine performance data is normally presented to the owner in the form of graphs. Against engine revolutions the gross power output is shown; and sometimes the net shaft power output (including reduction gearbox).

The propeller law curve shows the power which the propeller is capable of absorbing at different engine speeds. It is assumed that the correct propeller is fitted to allow the engine to reach its maximum revolutions at full throttle thus absorbing the full power that the engine is capable of developing. As the throttle is closed, the revolutions fall until idling speed is reached; the power decreases along the propeller law curve, not the full power curve. The propeller law curve depends on the exact matching of the propeller and hull form and is only provided in engine performance data as an arbitrary approximation. The torque curve should be fairly flat showing that the engine produces an even torque (engine turning power) throughout its power range.

In practice the engine performance data is of limited use except at full power. As the engine slows, the propeller is less efficient. Larger vessels have controllable pitch propellers to improve efficiency, but these are not practical on small craft. Boat performance also depends on the amount of fuel remaining, the cleanliness of the hull underwater and the sea state.

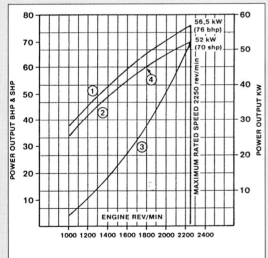

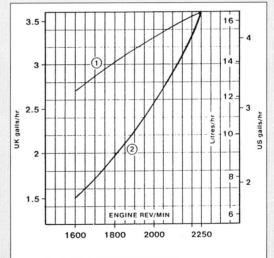

Rating Standard: BS Au141a:1971

1 Gross Power Output – engine without transmission.
2 Net Shaft Power (typical).
3 Propeller law curve (2.8 Index).
4 Minimum allowable rated speed for propeller matching.

Engine as delivered from factory will be set to produce gross power output within manufacturing tolerance and run-in allowance.

1 Full load fuel consumption.
2 Fuel consumption based on propeller law curve (2.8 Index) with propeller matched to full load rated speed.

4HD76 76 bhp (56,5kW)

Perkins

empty, so make sure that there are adequate baffles (see below) in the fuel tanks.

FUEL TANKS

The design of fuel tanks is important, particularly with diesel fuel where any aeration can have a disastrous effect on the engine. In a flat fuel tank, rolling up to 15° can reduce the effective size of the tank by 45%. This reduction can be minimised by fitting baffles to slow down the movement of fuel within the tank. In rough seas,when the fuel state is low and the fuel tanks do not contain sufficient baffles, it is possible for the fuel to roll to one side creating an airlock which could cause an engine malfunction and possible failure.

Suction should be taken from the middle of the tank. A V-shaped bottom to the tank is ideal. Over time, water and sludge collects in fuel tanks. Sludge traps and water drains are of equal importance to fuel filtration systems.

Ensure that all fuel tanks are thoroughly cleaned out and all fuel filters are replaced at least once every year.

It is no simple matter to calculate the effective fuel capacity of a boat, even when making no allowances for rolling and sloshing in a seaway. When calculating the cruising range of a boat, it is normal to assume that only 80% of normal fuel capacity is available. It is sensible to plan a passage to arrive with at least 25% fuel remaining. Fuel guages are usually hopelessly inadequate and although accurate gauges are available they are expensive. Sight glasses are cheap, simple and reliable; though some safety authorities (British Waterways and Thames Water) regard them as a fire and pollution hazard should the glass be shattered

QUESTIONS

3.1   You are looking at some motor cruisers at a Boat Show. One is fitted with twin Sabre 320L engines (developing 320 horsepower each), has a displacement of 16 tons, and a waterline length of 49 ft. What maximum speed would you expect it to achieve?

3.2   A fishing friend of yours has a displacement craft of 60 ft waterline length and a displacement of 34 tons which needs a new engine. He is considering a Perkins 4HD76 diesel engine. What is the maximum speed that you would expect for his craft?

3.3   Using the fuel consumption curves for a planing craft (Fig 3.9) and assuming a 400 litre fuel capacity but allowing for 90 litres of unusable fuel and contingency, work out a table to show how far the boat can go on the fuel remaining.

COMPASSES, CHARTS AND TIDES

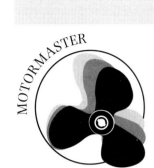

CHAPTER FOUR

COMPASSES

Unless you are cruising in rivers, an accurate compass is an essential piece of kit for any motorboater. You may only intend to cruise in sight of land, but sea mists and fog can materialise so fast, even in summer, that you can find yourself lost half a mile off shore. This is very unnerving if you are unprepared, and can put you and your boat in danger.

Once you decide to cruise further down the coast and need to plot a course on a chart, the compass is needed to provide accurate directional information.

Your boat may already be fitted with a compass of some sort but it may not be entirely suitable or it may require the attention of a compass adjuster (see page 17).

TYPES OF COMPASS

Card type compass

A card type compass consists of a transparent bowl filled with liquid, containing a graduated card mounted on a pivot. Attached to the card are magnets which provide a north seeking force. The north point of the compass card will point to magnetic north unless it is affected by other magnetic fields.

This type of compass works well at slower speeds but it is sensitive and can swing rapidly on fast-moving boats. When it is subjected to prolonged pitching and rolling the moving parts wear and the compass becomes unreliable. In such unstable conditions, it is not easy to read.

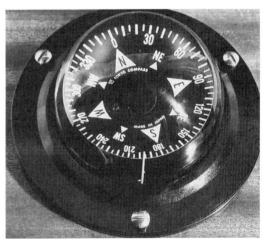

Card type compass. By courtesy of Yachting Instruments Ltd.

Installation

The compass needs to be installed on or parallel to the boat's longitudinal centre line, well away from ferrous metals, magnetic and electrical equipment and away from areas where there is much vibration. It should be in a position where the helmsman can read it easily.

After installation, the compass is corrected to remove as much deviation as possible (see page 17). The remaining small amounts of deviation are tabulated for various headings on the boat's deviation card or table (Fig 4.4).

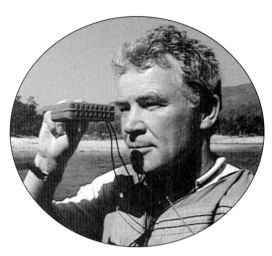

Using a hand-bearing compass

Hand-bearing compass

In addition to the boat's fixed compass you will also need a hand–bearing compass which is used to establish the boat's position by visual reference to landmarks (such as lighthouses) and seamarks (such as buoys). This small, easily portable magnetic compass can be used from any position on the boat. The direction of a mark as determined with a hand-bearing compass is known as a bearing (see Chapter 11).

A hand-bearing compass is also used to determine whether there is a risk of collision with an approaching vessel. A series of bearings is taken of the other vessel; if these bearings remain constant, then there is a risk of collision (see Chapter 23).

The use of a hand-bearing compass at speeds greater than 15 knots in even moderate seas is virtually impossible. If you need to confirm the position using visual bearings, then slow the boat down to less than 10 knots.

Electronic compass

An electronic or fluxgate compass consists of a heading sensor which measures the earth's magnetic field electronically, and one or more remote displays fed from the heading sensor. This is more suitable for use on a motorboat than the card type compass as there are no rotating parts or swinging cards.

The remote display can be either digital and include an off course steering indicator or digital with compass points. This type of compass will probably have a built-in automatic deviation compensator so it may never need adjusting.

Installation

The sensor can be located virtually anywhere in the boat but should be kept away from ferrous metal or objects which have strong magnetic fields, especially those which could move as the boat rolls, such as a toolbox. If there is anything seriously affecting the accuracy of the sensor, such as the close proximity of a magnetic object, warning is given by a visual display and an audible bleep.

After installation, to compensate for deviation caused by the boat's magnetic field, the boat is steered in a circle through 360°. It is best to do this out of the effects of the tidal stream or current and on a calm day to avoid too much pitching and rolling. The time taken to complete this circle should be at least two minutes. When the circle has been completed and the compensation calculated, the display unit emits a series of short bleeps. The accuracy achieved is ±0.5°.

On some models it is possible to enter magnetic variation so that the display shows true north (see page 15).

Interface capability

The sensor can be used to provide heading information to instrument and charting systems such as Decca, GPS, Loran, radar, autopilot and plotter.

Monocular fluxgate compass

This is a hand held device which combines an electronic fluxgate compass, an electronic range-finder, a digital chronometer and a 5 × 30 monocular telescope. The Datascope Fluxgate Compass is shown on page 19.

COMPASS ERROR

As previously mentioned, a magnetic compass is subject to errors brought about by the earth's magnetic field (*variation*) and the boat's magnetic field (*deviation*).

Variation

The earth's magnetic field consists of force lines which converge at the magnetic north pole. The location of the *magnetic* north pole differs slightly from the *true* or geographical north pole. The difference in direction between the two is known as **variation**. Variation differs from place to place and, because the magnetic pole is not stationary, can change slightly from year to year. The direction of the magnetic pole can be either east or west of geographical north (see Fig 4.1).

This is easy to understand when you look at the **compass rose** on a chart (Fig 4.2). The outer circle represents the true compass giving geographical north while the inner circle shows magnetic north. The angle shown between the two poles is the variation.

Applying variation

The chart extract in Fig 4.2 is for an area in the English Channel between Weymouth and Cherbourg. The variation for that area was 6°W in 1991, decreasing about 5′ annually. By 1999 it will have decreased 40′, so variation will be 5°20′W, though in practice you would correct to

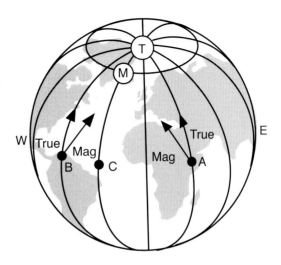

Fig 4.1 **Variation.** *Magnetic north **M** is off-set slightly from true north **T** so the variation between the two will depend on where you are on the Earth. At point **B**, variation is east; at **A** it is west. At **C** the variation is nil since true and magnetic north are directly in line.*

the nearest whole degree, 5°W.

A true course (T) or bearing, taken from a chart, is converted to a magnetic course (M) for steering by *adding* westerly or *subtracting* easterly variation.

Course	170° T (true)	Course	214° T
Variation	+ 6° W	Variation	− 8° E
Course	176° M	Course	206° M

When converting a magnetic course to true subtract westerly variation and add easterly variation.

There are many *aides-memoires* to help you to remember whether to add or subtract variation, probably the easiest is

Error West – compass best (**add**)
Error East – compass least (**subtract**)

MOTORMASTER

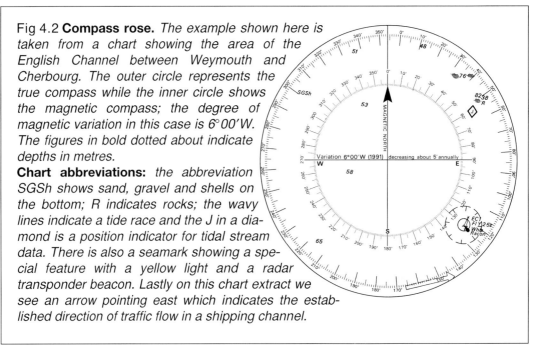

Fig 4.2 **Compass rose.** *The example shown here is taken from a chart showing the area of the English Channel between Weymouth and Cherbourg. The outer circle represents the true compass while the inner circle shows the magnetic compass; the degree of magnetic variation in this case is 6°00'W. The figures in bold dotted about indicate depths in metres.*

Chart abbreviations: *the abbreviation SGSh shows sand, gravel and shells on the bottom; R indicates rocks; the wavy lines indicate a tide race and the J in a diamond is a position indicator for tidal stream data. There is also a seamark showing a special feature with a yellow light and a radar transponder beacon. Lastly on this chart extract we see an arrow pointing east which indicates the established direction of traffic flow in a shipping channel.*

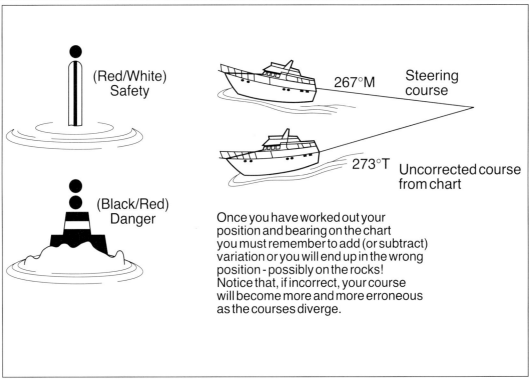

(Red/White) Safety

(Black/Red) Danger

267°M   Steering course

273°T   Uncorrected course from chart

Once you have worked out your position and bearing on the chart you must remember to add (or subtract) variation or you will end up in the wrong position - possibly on the rocks! Notice that, if incorrect, your course will become more and more erroneous as the courses diverge.

Fig 4.3 *Applying variation.*

MOTORMASTER

Deviation

Variation is not the only compass error that you have to consider. Deviation is another error to take into account. This is caused by the presence of ferrous metal, electrical and electronic equipment on your boat. When these are in close proximity to the compass they cause the compass needle to deviate east or west from magnetic north. So, what do you do about this? You will need to try to ensure that the compass is sited as far away as possible from electrical equipment and do not leave metal objects lying near it.

Compass adjustment

If you are worried about the accuracy of your compass, you can call in a compass adjuster. He or she will compensate for the error by adjusting the compass and prepare for you a deviation card (see Fig 4.4) because the deviation will vary according to your boat's heading.

Applying deviation

So now you know what the deviation is, how do you apply it? You use the same rule as for variation after you have applied the variation given on the chart. You can remember the order to apply variation and deviation errors by the CADET rule:

Compass → ADd   East → True

To convert a compass course to a true course, add easterly deviation/variation or subtract westerly deviation/variation. To work out the compass course, given a true course, the rule is applied in reverse:

Compass course	160° C	True course		314°T
Deviation	3°E+	Variation		4°W+
Magnetic course	163°M	Magnetic course	318°M
Variation	6°W-	Deviation		2°W+
True course	157°T	Compass course	320°C

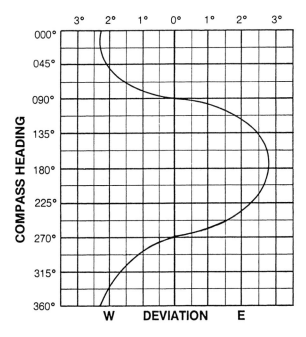

COMPASS HEADING	DEVIATION
000°	2½°W
020°	2½°W
040°	2°W
060°	2°W
080°	1°W
100°	1°E
120°	2°E
140°	2½°E
160°	3°E
180°	3°E
200°	2½°E
220°	2°½E
240°	1½°E
260°	½°E
280°	½°W
300°	1½°W
320°	2°W
340°	2°W

Fig 4.4 **Deviation card.** *The compass adjuster will give you a card with the deviation displayed as a graph (left). You can make this into a table for easy reference (right).*

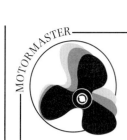

ELECTRONIC COMPASSES

This electronic digital compass has a memory to store the course you require as a reference heading.

The display (below) shows you how far off course you are from the latest reference heading. Degrees to port show up as segments on the left side of centre and degrees to starboard show up as segments on the right side. Plus or minus signs appear to show whether you are higher or lower than the reference heading.

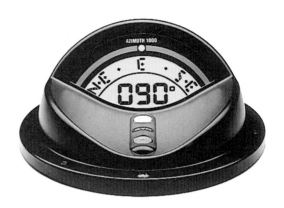

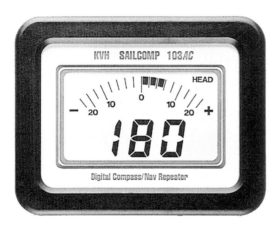

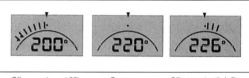

| Off course to port 20° | On course: Course = 220° | Off course to stbd. 6° |

In addition to giving a digital read-out of your heading, this electronic compass shows the familiar compass points. You can also lock on to a course which changes the compass rose to a steering indicator (below) that clearly shows when you are off course.

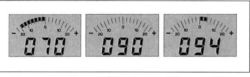

Off course to port 20°   On course: Course = 090°   Off course to stbd. 4°

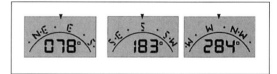

This compass type has selectable damping levels which enable you to adjust the compass read-out to the sea conditions; so even if the sea is rough or you are travelling fast, you will still have an accurate reading.

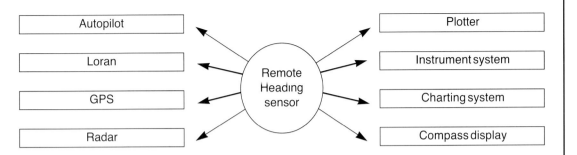

Autopilot		Plotter
Loran	Remote Heading sensor	Instrument system
GPS		Charting system
Radar		Compass display

Many electronic compasses can interface with your other onboard electronic position-finding equipment.

Hand-bearing compasses

Even the traditional magnetic hand-bearing compass now has its electronic counterpart in the form of the monocular fluxgate compass.

This combines compass, 5×30 monocular telescope with an electronic rangefinder in one unit. It has sufficient magnification to identify marks with ease and the range can be determined once the height is entered using a segmented scale. It is lightweight and requires only one hand to operate it. It makes easy work of bearing-taking accurately recording up to nine bearings and the times they were taken.

Compass Mode
The DataScope measures bearing with 0.1′ resolution at the touch of a button. The display indicates the bearing in memory No 2 is 325.8 ° which is roughly NW on the compass rose.

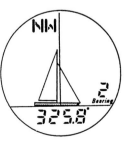

Range Mode
Once height is entered, matching the bar segment scale to the height of the target determines the distance. The lighthouse is approximately 1245 feet away.

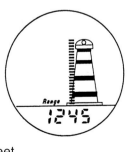

QUESTIONS

4.1   What influences affect a magnetic compass.

4.2   What is the variation in mid-Channel between the Cherbourg peninsula and the Isle of Wight for the year 1996? (See Fig 4.2)

4.3   a. Correct the following true bearings to magnetic bearings:

Bearing	Variation
218°T	6°W
147°T	4°E
359°T	10°W

b. Correct the following magnetic bearings to true bearings:

Bearing	Variation
001°M	9°W
178°M	7°E
007°M	5°E

4.4   a. Correct the following magnetic bearings to compass bearings:

Bearing	Deviation
010°M	9°E
356°M	8°W
162°M	4°E

b. Correct the following compass bearings to magnetic bearings:

Bearing	Deviation
241°C	10°W
054°C	12°E
292°C	3°W

4.5   A boat whose electronic compass has failed is using a standby card type compass. She is steering a mean course of 180°C. The variation is 6°W; the deviation is shown in deviation card Fig 4.4. The following bearings are taken:

Tower   091°C
Church   167°C
Monument   330°C

a. What are the true bearings?
b. What is the compass error?

4.6   What should be considered when siting an electronic compass?

MOTORMASTER

CHARTS

A chart is a sailor's equivalent of a road map. It will show conspicuous features on land and their names; seamarks and depths plus many other items of information. It will enable you to familiarise yourself with the area in which you want to cruise and to plan your best, safest route.

HOW IS A CHART DRAWN?

The object is to make a flat representation or projection of the Earth's curved surface.

There are several ways of doing this. The Mercator projection is most commonly used for navigational charts. It can be imagined as though a cylinder of paper encloses the Earth and touches the surface around the Equator. The image of the Earth's surface is projected on to the paper.

As you can see in Fig 5.1, the Earth is overlaid with imaginary lines of latitude and longitude. Lines of latitude, known as *parallels of latitude*, run parallel to the Equator north and south. Latitude is 0° at the Equator increasing to 90° at each pole.

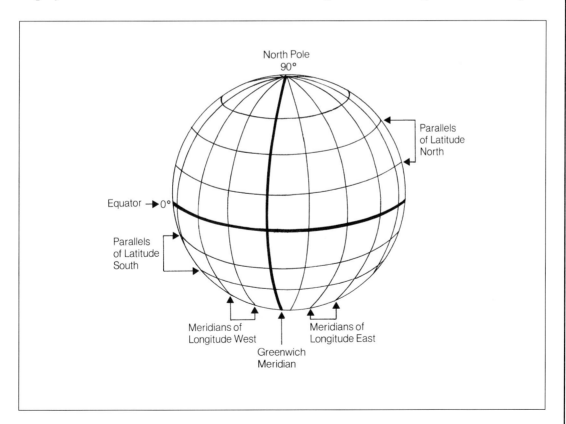

Fig 5.1 *Parallels of latitude and meridians of longitude.*

Lines of longitude, known as *meridians*, converge at the North and South Poles. The meridian passing through Greenwich, London, is known as the prime meridian, ie longitude 0°. Longitude is measured 0°–180° east and west of the Greenwich meridian. In a mercator projection, meridians appear as parallel lines at right angles to the parallels of latitude. To allow for the east-west distortion, the parallels of latitude are spaced increasingly further apart as the distance from the Equator increases. On this form of projection a straight line representing the track of a vessel crosses all meridians at the same angle. Such a line is known as a *rhumb line*. Because of the distortion of this projection, Mercator charts cannot be used either for polar regions (latitudes greater than 70°) or for passages in excess of 600 nautical miles. The charts in these cases use a *gnomonic* (or *Great Circle*) projection which shows meridians converging towards the Poles. A gnomonic projection equates to a flat sheet of paper touching the Earth's surface at a single point: commonly the North or South Poles. A straight line drawn on a gnomonic chart is called a *great* circle – the shortest distance between two points on the Earth's surface. For convenience, large scale charts use a gnomonic projection. For plotting purposes there is no practical difference between large scale gnomonic projection and mercator projection.

Measurement scales

Both the latitude and longitude scales are divided into units called degrees (°) with sub-divisions into minutes (') and tenths of a minute. There are 60 minutes in one degree. Sixty degrees ten point five minutes would be written: 60° 10'.5. Like a grid, co-ordinates from both scales are used to identify a position. The latitude scale is also used for measuring distance because **one minute of latitude is equivalent to one nautical mile (M)** (see Fig 5.2).

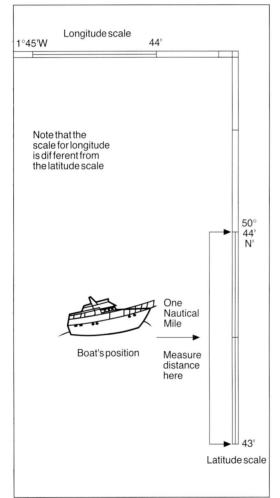

Fig 5.2 *Chart extract showing how to read off distance by using the latitude scale; one minute of latitude equals one nautical mile (M).*

WHAT DOES THE CHART SHOW?

Title and number

A chart is named according to the area which it covers. Fig 5.5 shows the title of a chart covering the western section of the English Channel. A chart also has a

CHART SCALE

Fig 5.3 shows a portion of a Stanfords chart which covers the area from the Needles, Isle of Wight, to Start Point. The title of the chart is: *The English Channel from the Needles to Start Point*; and the chart number is 12. It is a small scale chart showing a large area but not much detail and is used for planning a sea passage. Note Studland Bay on the left side of the chart. Now look at

Fig 5.4 which is a portion of Chart Number 15: *Poole Harbour and Approaches*. It is a larger scale than Chart 12. Studland Bay is shown in much more detail. This type of chart is used when approaching a harbour or an anchorage as it includes many of the features and hazards that are omitted on a small scale chart.

Fig 5.3 *A portion of Stanford's small scale Chart No 12 which shows the Western section of the English Channel.*

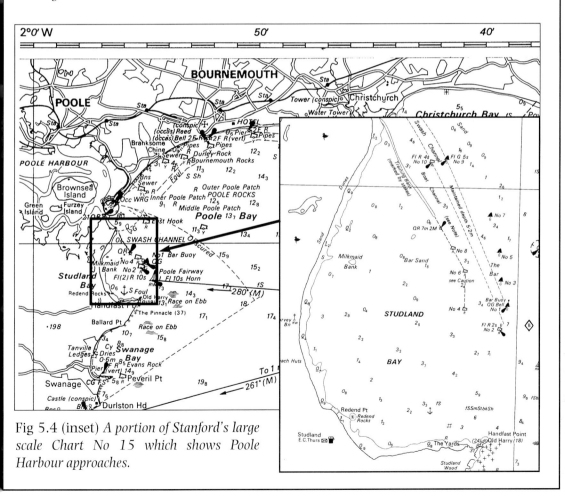

Fig 5.4 (inset) *A portion of Stanford's large scale Chart No 15 which shows Poole Harbour approaches.*

number printed in the corner and the title and number are also printed on the outside cover of the chart.

Units of measurement

Printed above the number in the corner of the chart are the words 'soundings in metres'. This means that all heights of land objects and depths of water are in metres, eg 3_7 is 3.7 metres. Calculation of these heights and depths will be based on the lowest astronomical tide; this reference level is known as *chart datum*. Areas which dry out show height above chart datum as an underlined figure. (See Fig 5.8).

Chart symbols

Below the title on Chart No 2, Fig 5.5, there is an explanation of some of the symbols used on the chart. Whilst such a key is included on some charts, generally you will have to refer to another publication, such as *Symbols and Abbreviations used on Admiralty Charts*, referred to as Chart 5011, published in booklet form. There is also a US publication *Nautical Chart Symbols and Abbreviations, Chart No 1*.

Chart symbols include buoys, lights, fog signals, anchorages, harbour entrances, hazards, wrecks and obstructions. Chapter 9 BUOYAGE gives examples of the most common chart symbols.

Tidal Streams referred to HW at PORTSMOUTH						
	Ⓐ	50°37'.0N 1 51 .0W		Ⓑ	50°39'.2N 1 54 .9W	
		Rate (kn)			Rate (kn)	
Hours	Dir	Sp	Np	Dir	Sp	Np
Before HW 6	053	1.3	0.6	344	1.4	0.7
5	049	2.0	1.0	346	1.2	0.6
4	057	2.1	1.0	354	1.0	0.5
3	053	1.9	1.0	004	0.7	0.3
2	046	1.3	0.6	029	0.3	0.2
1	103	0.3	0.1	157	0.3	0.1
HW	242	1.2	0.6	179	0.8	0.4
After HW 1	238	2.3	1.1	180	1.1	0.5
2	231	2.3	1.2	178	1.2	0.6
3	232	2.0	1.0	172	1.1	0.6
4	229	1.2	0.6	156	0.6	0.3
5	225	0.1	0.1	026	0.3	0.1
6	053	1.0	0.5	347	1.2	0.6

Fig 5.6 *Tidal stream information is given as a table on the chart. The areas covered by the table are given on the chart as a letter within a diamond shape: tidal diamonds.*

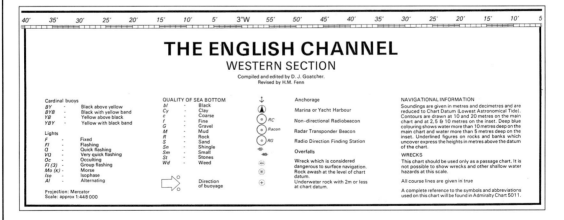

Fig 5.5 *The title of Stanfords Chart No 12 which gives some abbreviations, symbols and navigation information.*

MOTORMASTER

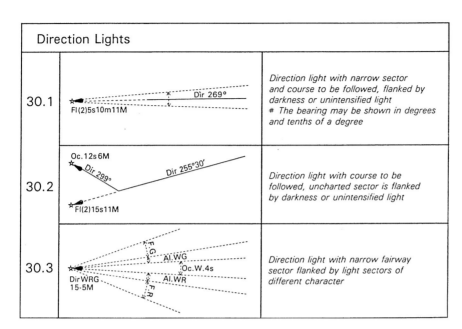

Tidal streams

Tidal stream information is shown in a table as in Fig 5.6. On charts, tidal streams are represented as a letter within a diamond (see Fig 5.4). For the area just off Studland Bay you would use tidal diamond B. You use the information to work out the direction and speed of tidal flow (see Chapter 7.)

Compass rose

When we looked at compass variation in Chapter 4 we saw that the compass rose (Fig 4.2) enables us to find the correct direction; on each chart there is at least one compass rose. Geographical or true north is indicated on this circular scale by 0° on the outer scale, east by 90°, south by 180° and west by 270°.

Depth contours

A line joining points on the seabed of equal depth is known as a contour line (see Fig 5.8). In areas where these contours are

fairly straight they can be used to keep a safe distance offshore.

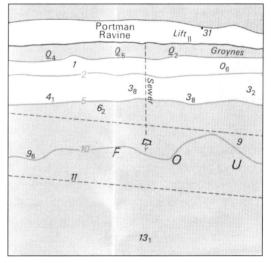

Fig 5.8 *Part of a chart showing Poole Bay where you can see three depth contour lines: 2, 5 and 10 metres. The closeness of the lines indicates fairly steep shelving from the beach. By the shore there is an area which dries out: drying heights are shown underlined eg $\underline{0_5}$ dries to a height of 0.5 metres above chart datum.*

Cautions

These are warnings of particular hazards which must be read before using the chart:

> **CAUTION**
> The buoys in Poole Harbour and approaches may be moved to meet changes in the channels. The minor channels are marked by stakes painted green with cone topmarks on the starboard–hand and red with can topmarks on the port–hand side.
>
> **SMALL CRAFT CHANNEL**
> This channel has been established for use by recreational craft with draughts of up to 1.5 metres. Such vessels should use the channel whenever possible.

Pilotage information

On the reverse of some charts, you will find navigation and pilotage information:

> Hengistbury Head is 18 metres high: a stone groyne extends for one cable south from the headland and its southern extremity is marked by a beacon. Beerpan Rocks lie half a cable south of this beacon.
>   Christchurch Ledge extends two and three quarter miles south east from Hengistbury Head with depths of five metres over it within one and a quarter miles of the coast. Overfalls can develop over the ledge on the ebb at springs.

CHART PUBLISHERS

In the United Kingdom, charts are published by the Hydrographer of the Navy (called Admiralty charts), and by two private firms, Imray, Laurie, Norie and Wilson who produce Imray charts, and Stanfords who produce Stanfords charts. You can buy these at most good chandlers and they are all available from chart agents who have catalogues listing charts by name and number. In the USA charts are published by various authorities two of which are The Defense Mapping Agency and The National Oceanic and Atmospheric Administration, National Ocean Service.

Many countries publish charts based upon information from their own hydrographic sources. It is worthwhile obtaining such local charts where possible as the information may have been from recent surveys.

CHART CORRECTION

For safe navigation, charts and related nautical publications must be corrected regularly in order to incorporate changes. The date to which a chart has been corrected is normally shown in the bottom left hand corner of the chart. Corrections for Admiralty charts are given in *Admiralty Notices to Mariners*, either the weekly edition covering charts worldwide, or the *Small Craft Edition* limited to northwest Europe. Private firms publishing charts usually offer a correction service by issuing amendment sheets periodically or charts can be returned to them.

Admiralty Notices to Mariners

For the correction of Admiralty charts, this publication contains notices numbered in sequence throughout the year, listing affected charts and giving the correction and number of the previous notice affecting the same chart. When a chart has been corrected, the number of the notice concerned is inserted in the bottom left hand margin so that a check can be made that no corrections are missing.

Where the corrections are difficult to do by hand, a small facsimile stick-on portion is provided. Important changes are promulgated immediately as navigational warnings by Coast Radio Stations. These are collected and issued in the weekly editions of *Admiralty Notices to Mariners*. Temporary changes and details of provisional changes are suffixed with a T or P respectively.

If corrections are extensive a new edition of the chart is published, announced beforehand in *Admiralty Notices to Mariners*. The date of the new edition is printed in the bottom margin immediately after the date of the original publication.

Admiralty Notices to Mariners Annual Summary is published by the Hydrographic Office and is available in January from Mercantile Marine Offices, Customs Houses and chart agents. It includes information on distress and rescue, warnings by Coast Radio Stations, details of firing practice and exercise areas and other items of interest to larger shipping. The weekly edition contains mainly chart corrections and is also available from the same sources.

Small Craft Edition

A Small Craft Edition available at chart agents is issued four times a year and contains a summary of the corrections to home waters charts and associated publications.

QUESTIONS

Use the chart extracts in this chapter to answer these questions.

5.1   What is the main difference between the portions of Chart No 15 and Chart No 12 (Figs 5.3 and 5.4)?

5.2   What is the title of Chart No 12 (Fig 5.5)?

5.3   What are the figures along the top of the chart (Fig 5.3)?

5.4   How can a specific position be identified on Chart 12?

5.5   What are the properties of a Mercator projection chart?

5.6   Why is it not possible to use Mercator projection charts for polar regions and for passages over 600 nautical miles?

5.7   What is the prime meridian for longitude?

5.8   What publication shows chart symbols and abbreviations?

5.9   How are charts corrected to date?

5.10   How would you write in figures: Fifty degrees, thirty eight point five minutes?

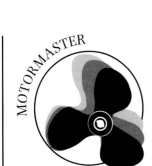

CHAPTER SIX

USING A CHART

Your new boat may be equipped with sophisticated electronic navigation equipment and you may wonder why you need to know how to work out your position on a paper chart. Imagine yourself setting off to Cherbourg from Dover; you are half-way there and your electronics go down due to a power failure. If you don't know the basics of chartwork you are effectively lost. That will never happen, you think, but wouldn't you feel safer and more confident knowing that should electronic failure occur, you can at least roughly work out where you are and in what direction to steer? In addition, if you are planning to take your cruiser abroad, there are some European countries which require a certificate of competence to visit their waters. As an answer to this the RYA devised the International Certificate of Competence which has practical and theory tests. The latter requires mastery of basic navigation skills using chartwork, so get out a chart and have a go at plotting – it's not as difficult as you may think.

PLOTTING INSTRUMENTS

For working on charts, you will need instruments to draw straight lines and to measure direction and distance:

Pencils and erasers A soft-leaded pencil (2B) will leave a strong black line on the chart and can be easily rubbed out with a good eraser.

Plotters Parallel rules or protractors can be used to measure direction but the most user-friendly instrument is the Breton plotter, Fig 6.1, sold by most chandlery shops. It consists of a plastic rectangle with its own integral rotating compass rose. A bearing can be very easily set by aligning the grid on the rose with a meridian on the chart. The plotter also takes account of the variation when you convert from magnetic to true. The straight edge of the plotter is used to draw in the course.

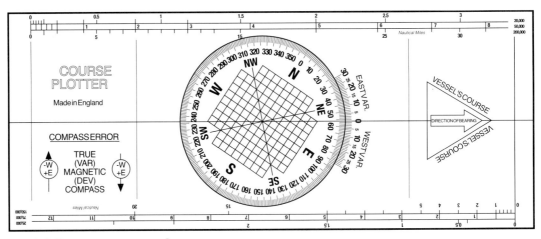

Fig 6.1 *Breton type course plotter.*

Dividers The best way of measuring distance along your course line is with a pair of brass dividers (at least 8 in (20 cm)).

When to plot

All your plotting should be done before you set off; once on passage, vibration and movement may make it impossible to plot positions or make any measurements on the chart. Generally charts should remain on or in the chart table and not be folded up or taken on deck, because they can blow away or be damaged by spray. Relevant navigational information needed for the passage should be entered in a notebook; the chart and pilot can then be used for reference. If there is doubt about the position of the boat, reduce your speed until the exact position can be properly determined.

To measure latitude

Using Fig 6.2, let us find the latitude of the red bell buoy in Start Bay. Place one point of the dividers on the buoy and the other point on the nearest parallel of latitude, which is 50° 20′N. Keeping them the same distance apart, transfer the dividers to the latitude scale, place one point on 50° 20′N and the other point will indicate the latitude of the buoy which is 50° 16.2′N.

To measure longitude

Look at Fig 6.3. The longitude of the buoy is measured in a similar way by using the meridian 3° 30′W and the longitude scale. The longitude of the buoy is 3° 33.9′W.

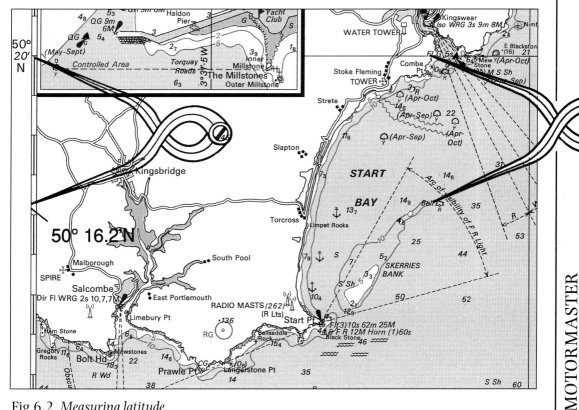

Fig 6.2 *Measuring latitude.*

MOTORMASTER

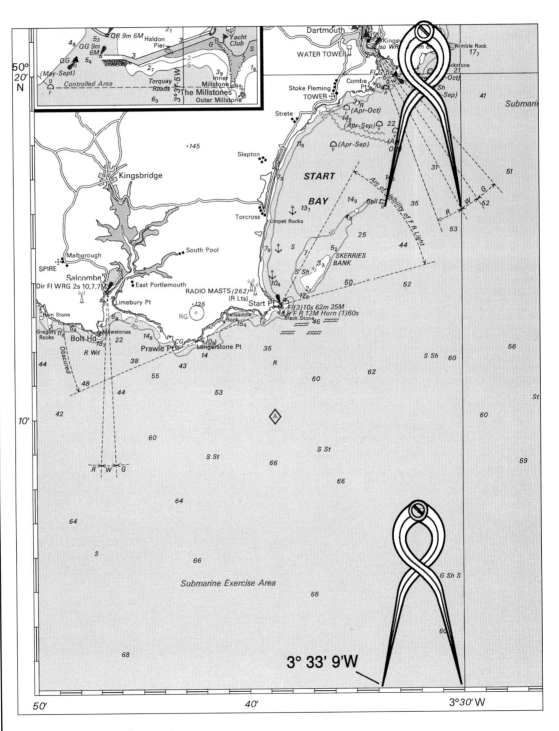

Fig 6.3 *Measuring longitude.*

Plotting a position

Now, suppose you have been given a position: 50° 08′N 3° 37′W and you want to find out where it is on the chart. It is the reverse of what you have just done. Dividers can be used to plot the latitude and longitude as shown in Fig 6.3. Note, when recording a position, latitude is written first followed by longitude.

Alternatively a course plotter can be used to plot latitude and dividers for longitude, Fig 6.4. Align the grid on the plotter so that the N–S line is across the plotter. Place one of the vertical grid lines on meridian of longitude 3° 30′W so that the edge of the plotter passes through the latitude scale at 50° 08′N. Leave the plotter in position. Use the dividers to find longitude 3° 37′W along the bottom scale using meridian of longitude 3° 30′W as a reference line. Move the dividers to the plotter and mark the position as shown in Fig 6.4.

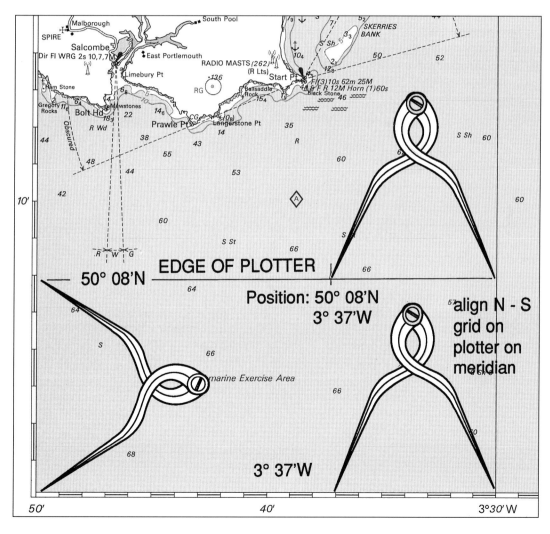

Fig 6.4 *Plotting a position using dividers and plotter.*

Finding direction

See Fig 6.5. You may want to know the direction from tidal diamond A to tidal diamond B. Place the edge of the plotter so that it passes through both points. Rotate the compass rose on the plotter until the N is upwards and align one of the vertical lines on the grid with a vertical line (meridian) on the chart. Read off the direction in line with the figure 0 on the outer edge of the compass rose. The direction is 056° True. (See explanation of magnetic variation in Chapter 6).

Plotting a direction

You may wish to travel in the direction 280°T. Using the plotter, line up 280° on the compass rose with 0° on the plotter. Keeping the rose fixed, place the edge of the plotter on position A and rotate the whole plotter until the N–S line on the grid comes in line with a meridian. Draw the required direction along the rule. Tidal stream can be plotted in the same way.

Plotting a bearing

You may wish to plot a bearing of 050°T. Line up 050° on the compass rose with the figure 0° on the plotter. Keeping the rose fixed, align the N–S line on the grid with a convenient meridian on the chart and at the same time align the edge of the rule on the chosen mark. Draw a line from the mark.

Measuring distance

Distance is measured in nautical miles. The latitude scale is used for measuring distance because one minute of latitude is equivalent to one nautical mile (abbreviated to M on charts). A nautical mile equals 1.15 statute miles.

On a chart, the size of the latitude scale can vary slightly so distance must *always* be measured from the latitude scale level with the boat's position. See Fig 6.6.

Fig 6.5 *Finding direction on a chart by using a course plotter.*

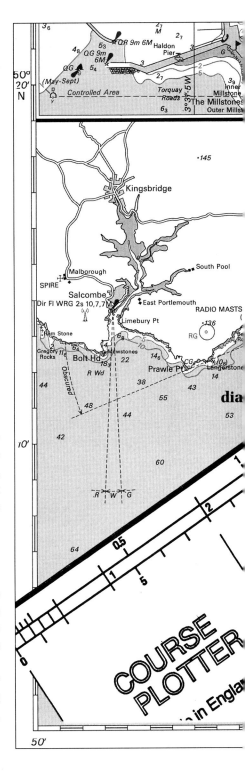

MOTORMASTER

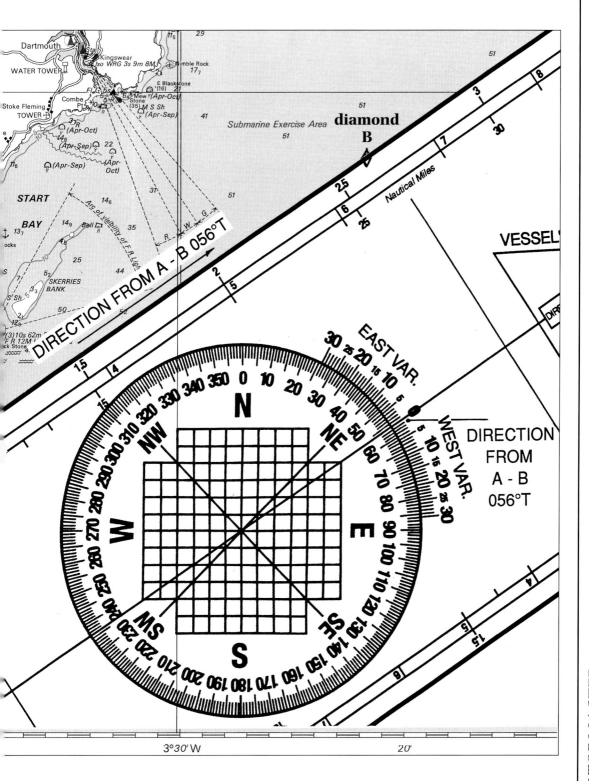

Dartmouth

Kingswear

Iso WRG 3s 9m 8M

WATER TOWER

Nimble Rock

17₇

Combe
Pt

E Blackstone
*(16)

Mew
Stone

(35) M S Sh

(Apr-Oct)

21

(Apr-Sep)

Stoke Fleming
TOWER

3₇
R
(Apr-Oct)

14₆
(Apr-Sep)

22

(Apr-
Oct)

11₆

(Apr-Sep)

START

BAY

14₆

14₉

Bell

R

35

13₇

25

31

Submarine Exercise Area

diamond
B

51

41

51

51

SKERRIES
BANK

44

50

52

Nautical Miles

DIRECTION FROM A - B 056°T

29

11₅

51

51

8

3

30

7

25

6

20

2

5

1·5

4

EAST VAR.

30 25 20 15 10 5

WEST VAR.

5 10 15 20 25 30

DIRECTION
FROM
A - B
056°T

VESSEL'

N

NW

NE

W

E

SW

SE

S

3°30′W

20′

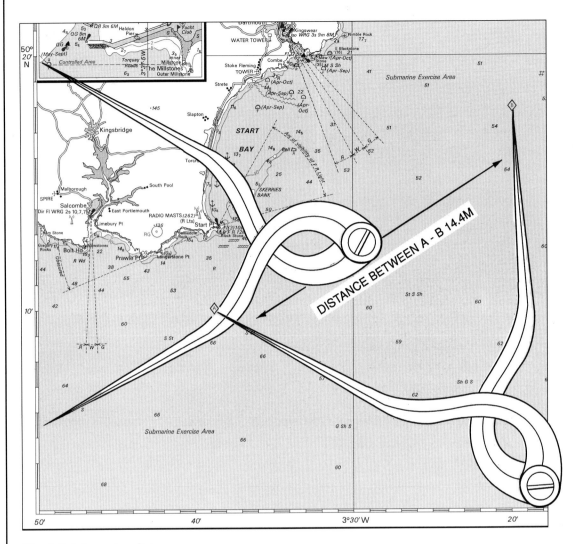

Fig 6.6 *Measuring distance.*

Let us measure the distance between tidal diamonds A and B. Open out the dividers and place the points on A and B. Keeping the points this distance apart, place them on the latitude scale level with the area covered by A and B. The number of minutes of latitude between the points of the dividers is 14.4, so the distance between A and B is 14.4 nautical miles which would be written 14.4M.

When measuring distances or marking tracks on a large scale chart, it is often convenient to fold over the edge of the chart so that it passes through both positions. The edge can now be used to draw the track line.

Defining position

A position is defined either by its latitude and longitude, or by its bearing and distance *from* a known landmark. The position of the red buoy in Figs 6.2 and 6.3 could be defined as 50° 16.2′N 3° 33.9′W or 045°T from Start Point light, 4.0 miles off, written 045°T Start Point light 4.0M.

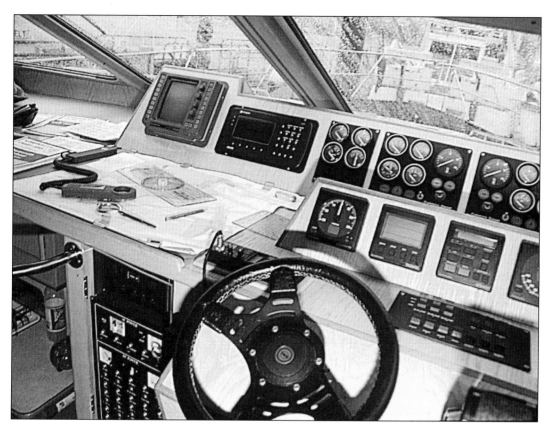

The cockpit of this motorcruiser has, beside the impressive display of instruments, a sizeable, well-equipped chart table.

QUESTIONS

Use the chart extracts in this chapter to answer these questions. Positions are shown to an accuracy of one tenth of a minute.

6.1   Why is it important to measure distance from the latitude scale in the area of the boat's position?

6.2   Using Fig 6.7, plot a position 50° 35.5′N 1° 57.5′W. What is in this position?

6.3   What is the latitude and longitude of the anchorage marked with a circle in Fig 6.7?

6.4   What is the latitude and longitude of a position 111°T from the flagstaff (*FS*) on Peveril Point 1.1M (Fig 6.7)? (*Note*: The flagstaff is in position 50° 36.4′N 1° 56.6′W.)

A subsidiary channel to be used by recreational craft and fishing vessels with a draught of up to 3.0m has been established on the western side of the Swash Channel. Such vessels should use this channel whenever possible.

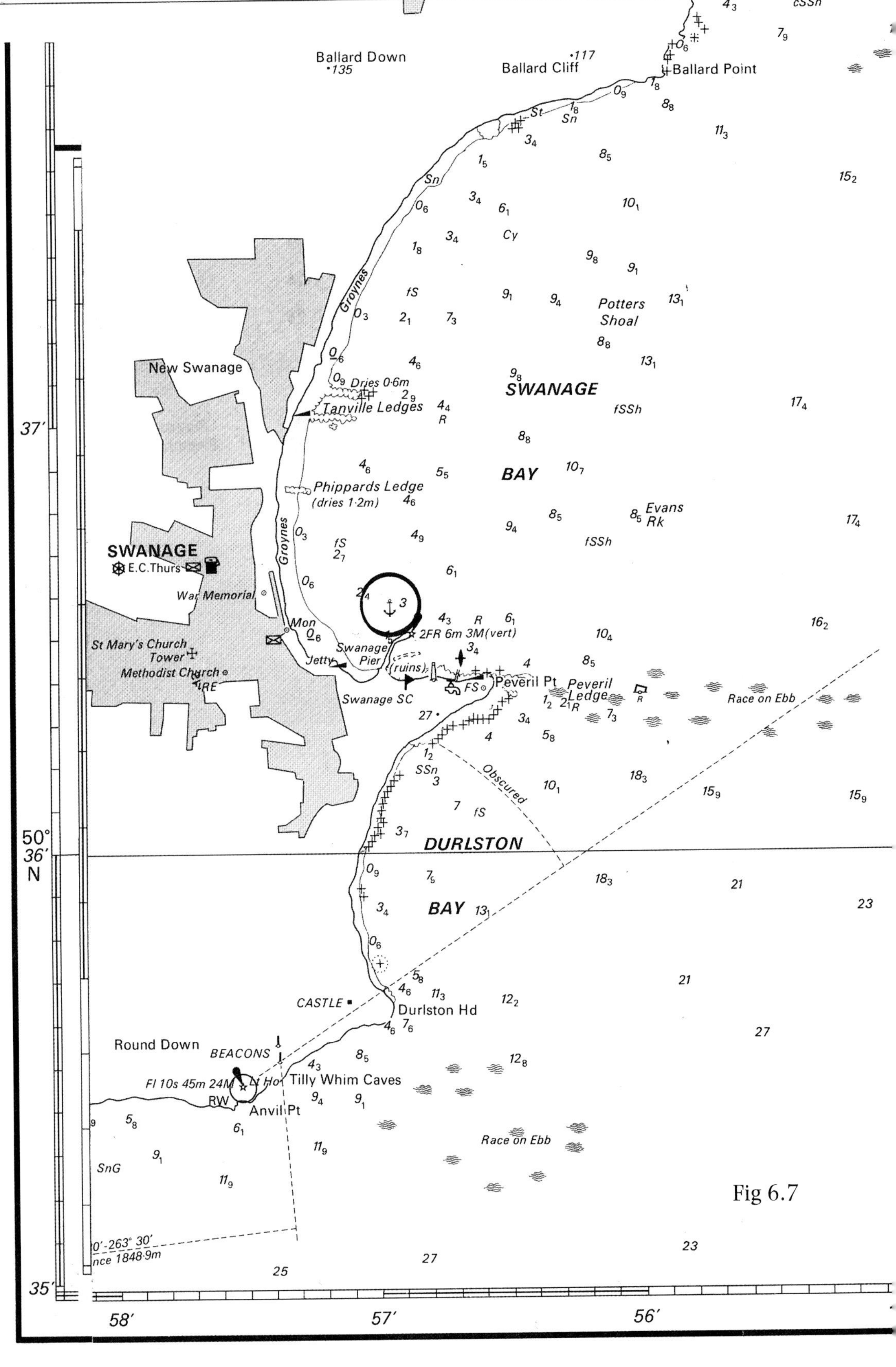

Ballard Down
•135

Ballard Cliff •117

Ballard Point

67•

cSSh

New Swanage

St. Sn

Sn

Groynes

Potters Shoal

SWANAGE

Dries 0·6m

Tanville Ledges
R

BAY

fSSh

Phippards Ledge
(dries 1·2m)

Evans Rk

fSSh

SWANAGE
E.C.Thurs

War Memorial

Mon

Groynes

St Mary's Church Tower
Methodist Church
RE

Swanage Pier
Jetty

(ruins)

☆2FR 6m 3M(vert)

Swanage SC

FS

Peveril Pt   Peveril
Ledge
R

Race on Ebb

27

SSn

Obscured

fS

DURLSTON

BAY

CASTLE

Durlston Hd

Round Down   BEACONS

Fl 10s 45m 24M   Lt Ho   Tilly Whim Caves
RW

Anvil Pt

Race on Ebb

SnG

Fig 6.7

0'-263° 30'
nce 1848·9m

37'

50°
36'
N

35'

58'   57'   56'

MOTORMASTER

6.5   Draw a line from the red buoy approximately 0.3M east of Peveril Point to a position 0.3M east off Ballard Point (Fig 6.7).
    a   What is the direction of this line?
    b   What is the distance between the red buoy off Peveril Point and the position off Ballard Point.
    c   What hazard is to the east of this line in the area of Ballard Point.

6.6   From the anchorage approximately 0.4M north west of Handfast Point (Fig 6.8):
    a   What is the direction of Poole Fairway buoy (50° 39′.O N 1° 54.8′W)?
    b   How far is it?
    c   If the boat speed is 8 knots, how long will it take to reach the buoy?

6.7   What does the symbol B to the north of Poole Fairway buoy mean (Fig 6.8)?

6.8   *a*   What is the bearing of Handfast Point from Poole Fairway buoy (Fig 6.8)?
    b   What is the distance?

Fig 6.8

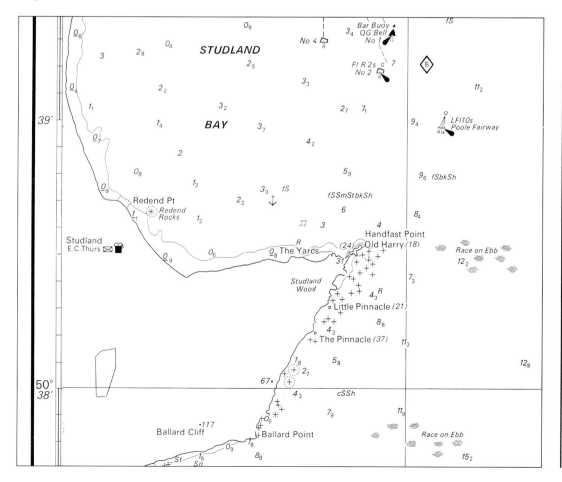

MOTORMASTER

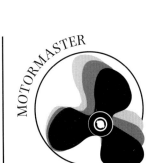

CHAPTER SEVEN

TIDES

Tides are vertical movements of water caused by a combination of the gravitational pull of the sun and the moon. Each day around the British Isles there are normally two high tides when the sea-level reaches its highest point, called *high water* (HW), and two low tides when the sea-level is at its lowest point, called *low water* (LW). A rising tide (flood tide) is the period between LW and HW, and a falling tide (ebb tide) the period from HW to LW.

The height difference between HW and the preceding or succeeding LW is called the *range*; and the time difference is called the *duration*. The difference from HW or LW to any given time is known as the *interval*.

The tide level does not rise and fall by the same amount each day. Over a period of approximately two weeks the heights of high water and low water vary from a minimum to a maximum then back to a minimum. The combination of the highest high water and the lowest low water (maximum range) is called a *spring* tide; and the combination of the lowest high water and the highest low water (minimum range) a *neap* tide (see Figs 7.1, 7.2 and 7.3). During one four week period there will be two spring tides and two neap tides.

At the time of the equinoxes (21 March and 23 September), when the earth and the sun are closest together, the spring tides have the greatest range and are known as *equinoctial spring tides*.

The height of a tide can be affected by weather conditions. If the barometric pressure is high (1040 millibars) over a period of several days, the increased pressure of the air on the sea surface can lower the sea-level by as much as 0.3 metres. A strong wind blowing into an estuary over a period of several days can raise the sea-level by a similar amount; or conversely lower it if the wind is blowing out to sea. Under these circumstances, variations in predicted heights and times of high and low water can occur.

CHART DATUM

Chart datum or *CD* is defined as the lowest level to which the tide is expected to fall due to astronomical conditions (Lowest Astronomical Tide or LAT). The depth of water shown on a chart (charted depth or *sounding*) is the depth of the seabed below chart datum. Other datum levels are shown in Fig 7.4. They are all 'mean' (average) levels taken over a period of one year: *mean high water springs* (MHWS) being the mean height above chart datum of the high waters of spring tides. Mean high water springs (MHWS) is used as the datum level for heights of land features. For comparison with the heights of land features shown on Ordnance Survey maps, large scale charts and tide tables include the differences between chart datum and the ordnance datum for various locations.

Drying height is the height that a rock or sandbar (normally covered at HW) projects above chart datum. *Height of tide* is measured from chart datum. *Depths* are measured from *height* to sea bed. The *charted depth* is measured from chart datum to the sea bed. The *height of lights* are measured from mean high water springs (MHWS).

Fig 7.1 *Tides are produced by the effects of the gravitational pull of sun and moon. When sun and moon are in line there are spring tides (highest highs and lowest lows). When sun and moon are at right angles there are neap tides (lowest highs and highest lows). The cycle of planetary movement is about 28 days so the changes occur more or less on a weekly basis.*

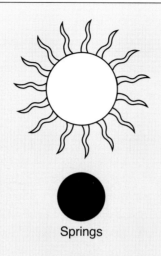

Springs

Neaps

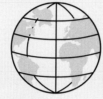

Neaps

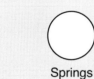

Springs

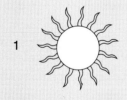

1

Spring tide

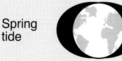

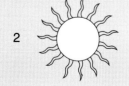

2

Fig 7.2 *1. When the moon and sun lie in a straight line with the Earth, their gravitational forces act in conjunction and result in a large rise and fall in sea level (spring tides).*
2. When the moon and sun form a right angle with the Earth, their combined effect is minimised, resulting in a smaller rise and fall in sea level (neap tides).

MOTORMASTER

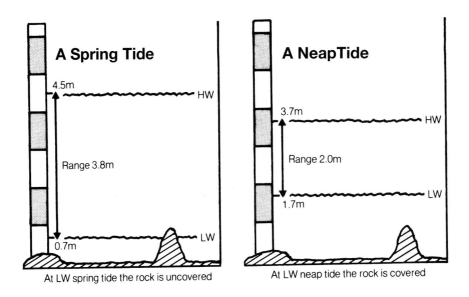

Fig 7.3 *Spring and neap tides.*

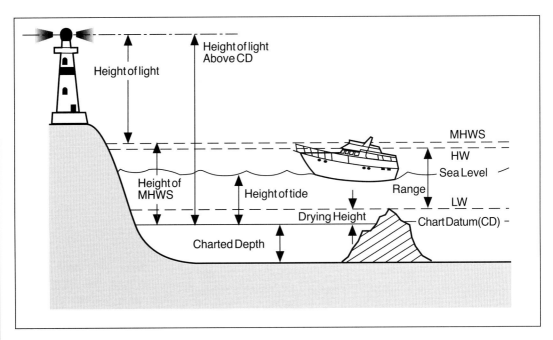

Fig 7.4 *Datum levels.*

TIDE TABLES

So how do we know what the height of tide will be at a certain time? We can find this information in Admiralty Tide Tables, a yachtsman's almanac or local tide tables (see Fig 7.6). These show the times and heights of high water and low water at main ports (called *standard ports*). For other ports, known as *secondary ports*, the times and heights of high water and low water are found by making corrections to the adjacent standard port times and heights. These corrections, known as *secondary port differences*, are found in a separate set of tables. Some local tide tables incorporate these differences.

The tables only give the height of the tide at the time of high water and low water. To find out the height of tide at times between high and low water, diagrams of *tidal curves* (Fig 7.5) are used. There are tidal curves given in almanacs

for each standard port; and, with certain exceptions, the same tidal curves are used for the associated secondary ports. The tidal curves also show the mean spring and neap ranges.

To understand how to use these tide tables and tidal curves let us work through some examples. All heights are in metres. All times are indicated using a four figure notation based on a 24 hour day, and are in local mean time (UK: Greenwich Mean Time[GMT]). During summer months one hour must be added (UK: British Summer Time [BST]).

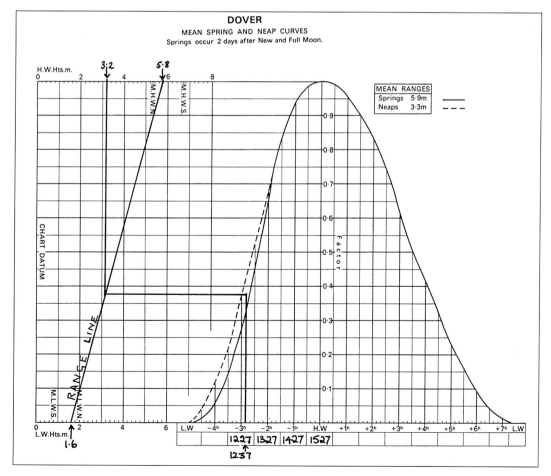

Fig 7.5 *Tidal curve diagram.*

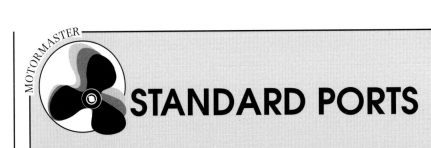

STANDARD PORTS

To find the time for a given height of tide at a standard port

Example: At what time (BST) at Dover during the afternoon of 2 June will the tide rise to a height of 3.2 m?

For the period covering the afternoon of 2 June, we look at the tide tables (Fig 7.6) for the port of Dover and take the time and height of high water (HW) and height of low water (LW). We then work out the range by subtracting the height of LW from the height of HW. We need to convert all the GMT times to BST.

	HW Time	*HW Height*	*LW Height*	*Range*
	1427 GMT	5.8 minus	1.6 =	4.2 (between neaps and springs)
Add one hour	+0100			
	1527 BST			

Now look at the tidal curve diagram in Fig 7.5.

1 On the time scale at the bottom of the tidal curve diagram fill in the time of HW (1527) and as we are looking for a time in the afternoon during the tide rise we need to fill in the hours in the boxes *before* 1527.

2 Now mark the height of HW (5.8) on the top height scale (HW Hts m) and the height of LW (1.6) on the bottom height scale (LW Hts m).

3 Draw the range line between the HW mark and the LW mark.

4 Mark the height of tide required (3.2) on the top height scale and draw a line vertically downwards to the range line.

5 From the point of intersection on the range line draw a horizontal line to the right to cut the rising (first) curve (if we were looking for a time on the falling tide you would run the line through to the second curve). Compare your range figure (4.2) with the mean ranges shown in the top right-hand corner of the tidal curve diagram: springs 5.9 m, neaps 3.3 m. In this case the range (4.2) is halfway (0.5) between the mean ranges for springs and neaps. So we need to *interpolate* (estimate) where the line ends; in this case half way between dotted line (neaps) and unbroken line (springs).

6 Draw a line vertically downwards from the tidal curve to the time scale and read off the interval: HW –2 hours 50 mins. Apply this interval to the time of HW to give the time required of **1237**.

(*Note*: An interval is shown as before or after HW by the use of a – or + sign.)

To find the height of tide at a given time at a standard port

Example: *What will be the height of tide at Dover on 17 May at 1100 BST?*

For the period including 1100 on 17 May, extract the time and height of high water and the height of low water from the tide tables for Dover and work out the range as we did in the previous example.

	HW Time	HW Height	LW Height		Range
	1341 GMT	6.2 minus	0.9	=	5.3 (near springs)
Add one hour	+0100				
	1441 BST				

Now look at the tidal curve diagram in Fig 7.7.
Proceed as for previous example as far as step 3.

4 Enter the time required on the time scale which is 3 hours 41 mins before HW (1100). Draw a line vertically upwards to the tidal curve interpolating between the spring and neap curves.

5 From this point on the tidal curve, draw a horizontal line to the left to the range line.

6 From the point of intersection on the range line draw a line vertically upwards to the height scale and read off the height which is **1.6 m**.

| | Lat. 51°07′N.   Long. 1°19′E. | **DOVER**
HIGH & LOW WATER |

MAY		JUNE		JULY		AUGUST	
Time m	Time m	Time m	Time m	Time m	Time m	Time m	Time m
1 0036 6·4 0757 0·9 F 1300 6·2 2006 1·1	**16** 0017 6·4 0745 0·8 Sa 1248 6·4 2008 0·9	**1** 0120 5·8 0840 1·4 M 1348 5·9 2101 1·5	**16** 0208 6·2 0934 1·0 Tu 1426 6·3 2159 0·9	**1** 0138 5·9 0857 1·5 W 1405 6·1 2121 1·4	**16** 0237 6·3 1013 1·0 Th 1450 6·4 2235 0·9	**1** 0223 5·9 0934 1·6 Sa 1442 6·1 2202 1·5	**16** 0335 5·9 1040 1·7 Su 1552 6·0 2313 1·7
2 0107 6·2 0827 1·1 Sa 1331 6·0 2042 1·3	**17** 0109 6·3 0833 0·9 Su 1341 6·2 2057 1·0	**2** 0157 5·6 0915 1·6 Tu 1427 5·8 2141 1·7	**17** 0300 6·1 1028 1·2 W 1517 6·1 2254 1·1	**2** 0219 5·7 0929 1·6 Th 1444 6·0 2159 1·5	**17** 0324 6·1 1052 1·3 F 1539 6·2 2319 1·2	**2** 0304 5·7 1010 1·7 Su 1524 5·9 2244 1·7	**17** 0431 5·5 1122 2·1 M 1654 5·6
3 0137 5·9 0901 1·4 Su 1405 5·8 2118 1·6	**18** 0206 6·0 0925 1·2 M 1434 6·0 2152 1·2	**3** 0242 5·4 0955 1·8 W 1515 5·6 2224 1·8	**18** 0356 5·9 1123 1·4 Th 1612 5·9 2353 1·2	**3** 0305 5·6 1006 1·8 F 1531 5·8 2240 1·7	**18** 0416 5·9 1134 1·6 Sa 1633 6·0	**3** 0356 5·5 1055 2·0 M 1620 5·5 2337 1·9	**18** 0546 5·2 Tu 1225 2·0 1819 5·2
4 0212 5·5 0938 1·7 M 1447 5·5	**19** 0307 5·8 1026 1·5 Tu 1531 5·8	**4** 0342 5·2 1041 2·0 Th 1614 5·5	**19** 0459 5·7 1221 1·5 F 1716 5·8	**4** 0400 5·5 1049 1·9 Sa 1624 5·7	**19** 0008 1·5 0516 5·6 Su 1224 1·9	**4** 0459 5·4 1158 2·2 Tu 1727 5·5	**19** 0126 2·4 0710 5·2 W 1359 2·5

Fig 7.6 *Extract from a Dover tide table.*

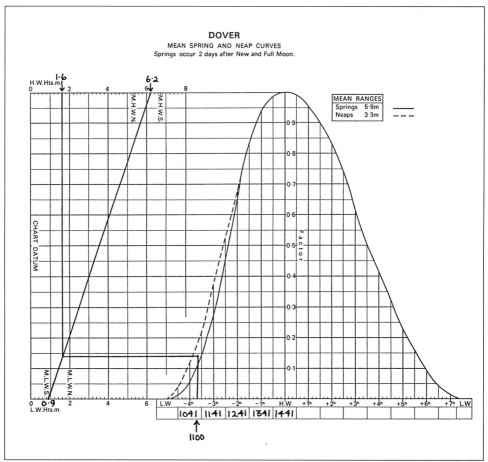

Fig 7.7 *Tidal curve diagram.*

Secondary ports

You can see that working out times and heights at standard ports using the tables and tidal curves is pretty straightforward but what if we are at a non-standard port? In your almanac or tide table you will find tables of *secondary port tidal differences* (Fig 7.8).

Suppose HW at Dover is at 0100 GMT and you wish to know the time of HW at Folkestone. Look at Fig 7.8; you will see that there are two columns for HW time differences and two for LW. The nearest figure to your time of 0100 is shown as **0000** in column one when the time difference for Folkestone is –20 minutes. At **0600** (column two) the time difference is –5 minutes. Therefore the range of difference is:

20 – 5 = 15 minutes

At 0100 you are one hour into the 6 hour interval so you need to find ⅙ of the range:

⅙ of 15 = ¹⁵⁄₆ = 2.5

	TIDAL DIFFERENCES ON DOVER							
	TIME DIFFERENCES				HEIGHT DIFFERENCES (Metres)			
PLACE	High Water		Low Water		MHWS	MHWN	MLWN	MLWS
DOVER	0000 and 1200	0600 and 1800	0100 and 1300	0700 and 1900	6.7	5.3	2.0	0.8
Hastings	0000	–0010	–0030	–0030	+0.8	+0.5	+0.1	–0.1
Rye (Approaches)	+0005	–0010	—	—	+1.0	+0.7	—	—
Rye (Harbour)	+0005	–0010	—	—	–1.4	–1.7	Dries	Dries
Dungeness	–0010	–0015	–0020	–0010	+1.0	+0.6	+0.4	+0.1
Folkestone	–0020	–0005	–0010	–0010	+0.4	+0.4	0.0	–0.1
Deal	+0010	+0020	+0010	+0005	–0.6	–0.3	0.0	0.0
Richborough	+0015	+0015	+0030	+0030	–3.4	–2.6	–1.7	–0.7
Ramsgate	+0020	+0020	–0007	–0007	–1.8	–1.5	–0.8	–0.4

NOTE: Rye should be carefully considered. It dries out, tidal streams are strong and rough weather can make Rye Bay very dangerous for small vessels.
Folkestone is unsuitable except in emergency.
Ramsgate is an excellent harbour for all small yachts.

Fig 7.8 *Extract from an almanac giving differences on Dover for some secondary ports.*

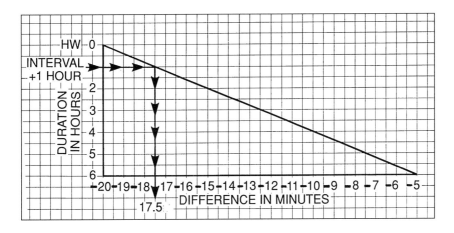

Fig 7.9 *A graphical solution for secondary port differences.*

Next take the 2.5 minutes (rounded to 3 for ease) from the first tabulated figure:

$$20 - 3 = 17 \text{ minutes.}$$

For a HW at Dover of 0100 GMT, the time difference for HW at Folkestone is minus 17 minutes. Take that from your time of 0100 and you now know that HW Folkestone is at 0043 GMT.

You might find it quicker and easier to work it out by using a graph (see Fig 7.9).

For height differences a similar interpolation is used.

To find the time that the tide will reach a given height at a secondary port

Example: At what time (BST) will the tide first fall to 2.5m at Ramsgate on 16 May?

For the period covering the falling tide on 16 May, extract the times and heights of high water and low water at the standard port, Dover (see Fig 7.6). Subtract LW heights from HW to work out the range, then (using **0000** as close enough) apply the tidal differences for the secondary port, Ramsgate (Fig 7.8).

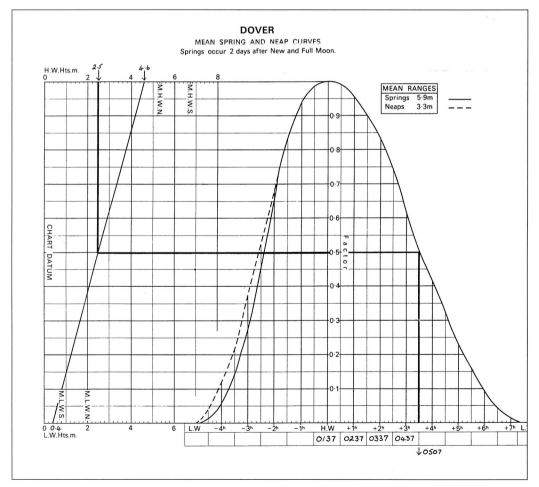

Fig 7.10 *Tidal curve diagram.*

	HW Time	HW Height (m)	LW Height (m)	Range
Dover	0017 GMT	6.4	0.8	5.6
Differences	+0020	−1.8	−0.4	(nearly springs)
Ramsgate	0037 GMT	4.6	0.4	
Add 1 hour	+0100			
Ramsgate	0137 BST			

Next look at the tidal curve diagram, Fig 7.10

The tidal curve diagram for the standard port is used but the times and heights of HW and LW at the secondary port are entered on the diagram. The range at the *standard* port is required for the interpolation between the spring and neap curves. The interval is HW + 3 hours 30 mins. The time required is **0507**. (Note that the time correction to BST is made after the differences for the secondary port have been applied.)

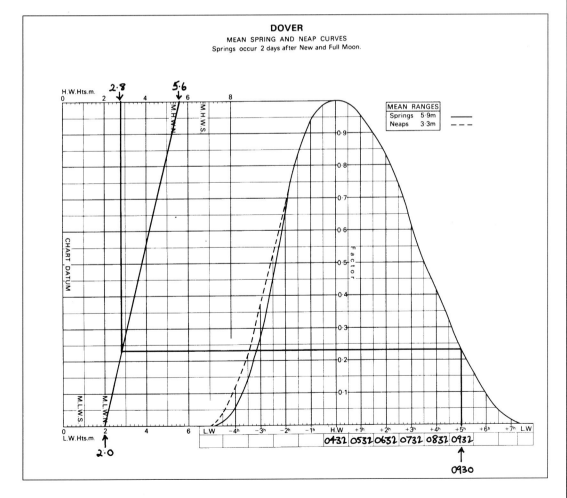

Fig 7.11 *Tidal curve diagram.*

To find the height of tide at a given time at a secondary port

Example: What will be the height of tide at Folkestone on 4 June at 0930 BST? Use Figs 7.6 and 7.8.

	Time	HW Height (m)	LW Height (m)	Range
Dover	0342 GMT	5.2	2.0	3.2 (neaps)
Differences	– 0010	+0.4	0.0	
	0332	5.6	2.0	
Add 1 hour	+0100			
Folkestone	0432 BST			

Look at the tidal curve diagram, Fig. 7.11. Height of tide: **2.8 m.**

SOLENT PORTS (SWANAGE TO SELSEY)

Look at Fig 7.12 which is the tidal curve diagram for Lymington and Yarmouth both of which come under the special classification of Solent ports. What are the differences between this diagram and the tidal curve diagram for Dover, Fig 7.5? There are two

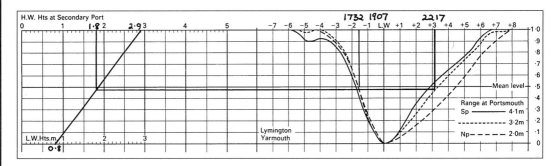

Fig 7.12 *Tidal curve diagram for a secondary port.*

differences: Lymington and Yarmouth are both secondary ports, the standard port for the area being Portsmouth; and the time intervals are from LW rather than HW.

In the area covered by the Solent ports the tides are complex with the result that HW can remain at a steady level (called a stand of the tide) or occasionally fall a little then rise again for a second HW. The tidal pattern varies considerably between ports adjacent to each other. Therefore it is easier to determine the time of LW rather than HW and so tidal curve diagrams use LW as the datum. As the tidal patterns of the secondary ports are so different from the standard port, Portsmouth, and from each other, a complete series of tidal curve diagrams is necessary. Poole Harbour, though not formally a standard port, has its own set of tide tables.

A slightly modified procedure is used with the tidal curve diagrams for Solent ports.

To find the time for a given height of tide at a Solent Port

Example: *At what time in the afternoon of 1 May will the tide at Lymington fall to a height of 1.8m?* (Use Figs 7.12, 7.13 and 7.14)

For the afternoon of 1 May, extract the time and height of LW and the height of HW for the standard port, Portsmouth, and apply the tidal differences from Lymington.

	HW	LW	LW	
	Height (m)	Time	Height (m)	Range
Portsmouth	4.4	1827 GMT	1.1	3.3
Differences	−1.5	−0020	−0.3	(mid range)
Lymington	2.9	1807 GMT	0.8	
Add 1 hour		+0100		
Lymington		1907 BST		

On Fig 7.12, fill in the time of LW and heights of HW and LW. Compare the range of tide at Portsmouth with the spring, neap and mid ranges shown on the tidal curve diagram to determine which curve to use. Proceed as for previous example for secondary ports.

Interval: LW −1 hour 35 mins. Time required **1732**.

PORTSMOUTH

HIGH & LOW WATER   **GMT** ADD 1 HOUR MARCH 29 – OCTOBER 25 FOR B.S.T.

MAY				JUNE				JULY				AUGUST			
TIME	M	TIME	M	TIME	M	TIME	M	TIME	M	TIME	M	TIME	M	TIME	M
1 0059	4.5	**16** 0047	4.7	**1** 0143	4.1	**16** 0213	4.4	**1** 0203	4.0	**16** 0248	4.5	**1** 0251	4.1	**16** 0356	4.2
0610	0.8	0606	0.6	0659	1.2	0739	0.8	0719	1.1	0815	0.8	0806	1.0	0919	1.4
F 1327	4.4	SA 1320	4.5	M 1423	4.1	TU 1503	4.5	W 1442	4.2	TH 1535	4.7	SA 1525	4.3	SU 1630	4.3
1827	1.1	1829	0.9	1919	1.6	2007	1.3	1941	1.5	2041	1.3	2027	1.3	2147	1.6
2 0131	4.4	**17** 0132	4.5	**2** 0220	4.0	**17** 0307	4.3	**2** 0240	4.0	**17** 0338	4.4	**2** 0330	4.1	**17** 0452	3.9
0642	0.9	0653	0.7	0738	1.3	0834	1.0	0756	1.2	0905	1.0	0847	1.2	1017	1.8
SA 1403	4.2	SU 1413	4.4	TU 1504	4.0	W 1602	4.5	TH 1520	4.2	F 1626	4.5	SU 1604	4.2	M 1727	4.0
1858	1.3	1917	1.1	2004	1.7	2105	1.4	2021	1.5	2133	1.4	2112	1.5	2254	1.8

Fig 7.13   *Extract from a tide table for Portsmouth.*

TIDAL DIFFERENCES ON PORTSMOUTH

PLACE	TIME DIFFERENCES				HEIGHT DIFFERENCES (Metres)			
	High Water		Low Water		MHWS	MHWN	MLWN	MLWS
PORTSMOUTH	0000 and 1200	0600 and 1800	0500 and 1700	1100 and 2300	4.7	3.8	1.8	0.6
Swanage	−0250	+0105	−0105	−0105	−2.7	−2.2	−0.7	−0.3
Bournemouth	−0240	+0055	−0050	−0030	−2.7	−2.2	−0.8	−0.3
Christchurch (Entrance)	−0230	+0030	−0035	−0035	−2.9	−2.4	−1.2	−0.3
Christchurch (Tuckton)	−0205	+0110	+0110	+0105	−3.0	−2.5	−1.0	+0.1
Hurst Point	−0115	−0005	−0030	−0025	−2.0	−1.5	−0.5	−0.1
Lymington	−0110	+0005	−0020	−0020	−1.7	−1.2	−0.5	−0.1
Bucklers Hard	−0040	−0010	+0010	−0010	−1.0	−0.8	−0.2	−0.3
Stansore Point	−0050	−0010	−0005	−0010	−0.9	−0.6	−0.2	0.0
Isle of Wight								
Yarmouth	−0105	+0005	−0025	−0030	−1.6	−1.3	−0.4	0.0

Fig 7.14   *Almanac extract giving differences on Portsmouth for some secondary ports.*

MOTORMASTER

To find the height of tide at a given time for a Solent Port

Example: What is the height of tide at Christchurch entrance on 16 July at 1140 BST?

	LW Time	LW Height (m)	HW Height (m)	Range
Portsmouth	0815 GMT	0.8	4.7	3.9
Differences	−0035	−0.4	−2.9	(spring)
Christchurch	0740 GMT	0.4	1.8	
Add 1 hour	+0100			
Christchurch	0840 BST			

Interval: LW +3 hours

Look at tidal curve diagram, Fig 7.15. Height of tide required: **1.5m**

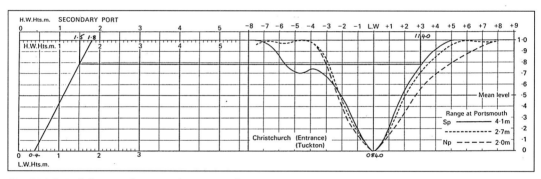

Fig 7.15 *Tidal curve diagram for a secondary port.*

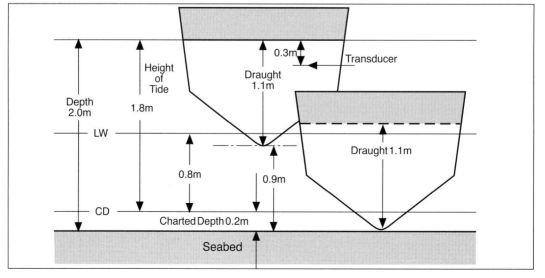

Fig 7.16   *At 1732 the boat has a clearance above the sea bed of 0.9 metres but at LW she will be aground.*

MOTORMASTER

Calculating depths of water

If you know the height of tide at a particular spot and look at the depths of water and drying heights shown on the chart you can work out the actual depth of water. If the draught of the boat is known, then the clearance between the bottom of the keel and the seabed can be worked out, Fig 7.16.

If the information on the chart is dubious or absent, use your echo sounder or lead line to estimate the charted depth. To allow for any rounding in the tidal calculations and for any abnormal weather conditions, a minimum clearance of 0.5 m between the hull and the seabed is normally assumed.

Example: In calm weather, a motorboat whose draught is 1.1 m anchors in the approaches to Lymington River at 1732 BST on 1 May. At that time the depth of water was 1.7 m as measured on the echo sounder which was sited 0.3 m below the waterline. Will she be aground at low water; and how much anchor chain should she let out if she intends to remain overnight?

Look at Fig 7.12.

Example on page 49 shows that the height of tide at Lymington at 1732 on 1 May is 1.8 m on a falling tide. LW is at 1907 and the height of tide at LW is 0.8 m. If the echo sounder is 0.3 m below the waterline and indicates 1.7 m, then the actual depth of water at 1732 is 2.0 m. The seabed is therefore 2.0 −1.8 = 0.2 m below chart datum (this means the charted depth would be shown as 0_2). The height of tide at LW is 0.8 m above chart datum or 0.8 + 0.2 = 1.0 m above the seabed. As the motorboat draws 1.1 m, **she will be aground at LW**. At the following HW the height of tide will be 2.9 m above chart datum or 2.9 + 0.2 = 3.1 m above the seabed. The rule of thumb to determine the length of anchor chain to let out is 4 × maximum depth of water or 4 × 3.1 = 12.4 m, so 13 m of anchor chain would be on the safe side. She has gone aground on a falling tide: by extending the horizontal line on Fig 7.12 across to the next rising tide, the time that she will refloat is LW + 3 hours 10 mins or 2217.

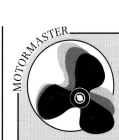

TIDAL DIAMONDS

Assessments of tidal streams are more important to yachtsmen than to motorboaters but there are areas, such as the Channel Islands where fierce tides can be encountered: the stream in Alderney Race can reach nearly 10 knots on a big spring tide – smaller engines will have a struggle against this. Also tidal calculations are an integral part of the chartwork which you will need to master to pass a navigation qualification such as the RYA Day Skipper and Yachtmaster certificates.

In the chart extract Fig 7.18 you can see tidal diamond K which covers the area south of the Isle of Wight. Beside the chart is an extract from the table on the chart (Fig 7.19) giving tidal stream information referring to HW Dover. On the table, the K symbol chart position is given: 50° 30.4'N and 1° 16.6'W. Below the K diamond the direction of the tidal stream is given as a true bearing. In the next column the rate in knots is given for springs and neaps. Down the side of the chart extract is a scale giving hours before and after HW. So if we are

two hours after HW (HW+2) the tidal stream for K will be setting (flowing) in the direction 276°T at a rate of 4.2 knots for springs and 2.1 knots for neaps.

But what if we are half-way between neaps and springs? Then we have to *interpolate* (estimate) between the rates given for neaps and springs. Looking at the tide table for the day in question we can then work out the range (HW minus LW); in this case we will take it as 5.1 metres. The standard range for Dover is 5.9 metres for springs and 3.3 metres for neaps. Now armed with this information we can plot a simple graph to estimate the rate:

◊ Begin the graph (Fig 7.20) by drawing in the range and rate scales.
◊ Mark the mean spring and neap ranges (5.9 m and 3.3 m) on the graph with horizontal lines.
◊ Using the rate scale, mark the tabulated neap rate at 2.1; mark the tabulated spring rate at 4.2.

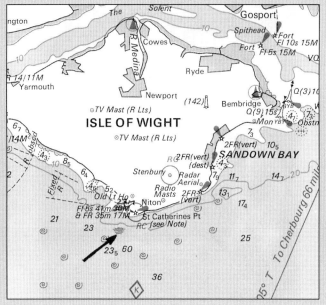

		50°16'N 1 48 W			50°30'·4N 1 16·6W			50°11'N 1 04 W	
Hours	Dir	Rate (kn) Sp	Np	Dir	Rate (kn) Sp	Np	Dir	Rate (kn) Sp	Np
Before HW 6	072	0·8	0·4	075	0·9	0·5	203	0·1	0·1
5	080	2·4	1·2	094	2·8	1·4	081	1·6	0·8
4	084	3·5	1·7	100	4·2	2·1	075	2·7	1·4
3	086	3·5	1·7	100	4·6	2·3	076	3·4	1·7
2	088	2·5	1·3	100	3·6	1·8	077	2·9	1·5
1	099	1·2	0·6	095	1·8	0·9	077	1·9	1·0
HW	238	0·7	0·4	320	0·4	0·2	107	0·5	0·2
After HW 1	263	2·3	1·1	276	2·6	1·3	254	0·8	0·4
2	270	3·4	1·7	276	4·2	2·1	276	2·2	1·1
3	266	3·3	1·6	276	4·2	2·1	260	3·1	1·5
4	265	2·6	1·3	276	3·4	1·7	250	3·6	1·8
5	265	1·5	0·7	285	1·8	0·9	254	2·9	1·4
6	040	0·2	0·1	005	0·4	0·2	249	1·1	0·6

Fig 7.18   *Chart extract (left) showing the Isle of Wight.*
Fig 7.19   *Extract (above) from a table giving tidal stream information.*

> Then draw an interpolation line diagonally between these two points.
> The range of 5.1 is drawn in as a horizontal line to intersect the interpolation line.
> Next, from the point of intersection, draw a line to the bottom rate scale which gives the rate, for a range of 5.1 as 3.5 knots. The direction is as given on the table: **276°T**.

If your boat was travelling on a westerly course (270°T) it would be assisted by the tidal stream which is flowing towards 276°T. In this case the tidal stream would be *fair*. But if the boat was travelling towards the east the passage time would be increased and the tidal stream would be *foul*. For a boat travelling north or south the tidal stream will be across the track and must be allowed for in determination of the course to steer. Later we will use the information from these tidal diamonds when we determine, by plotting on the chart, the effect of the tidal stream on the track of the boat.

The time scale

When working out tidal rates using the diamonds, you need to be aware that the directions of flow and rates given are each one hour of duration.

For example if HW Dover is at 1300 (springs) then looking at diamond K the times would work out at:

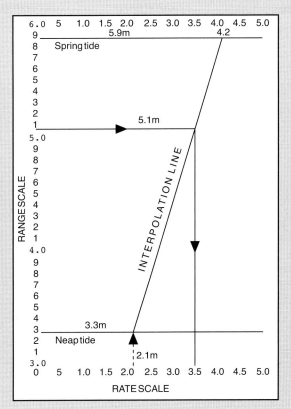

Fig 7.20 *Graph for interpolation between spring and neap rates.*

So from 0730 to 0830 the mean tidal stream would be 094° T 2.8 kn (HW −5). For the period from 0830 to 0930 the tidal stream would be 100° T 4.2 kn (HW −4). But if you wanted to know what the tidal stream would be from 0800 to 0900 then you have to take 30 minutes from HW −5 (094° T 1.4 M) and 30 minutes from that tabulated for HW −4 (100° T 2.1 M) (See note on page 97.)

The relevance of this will become plain when you plot your course on the chart (see Chapter 14).

	Dir	Rate Sp	(knots) Np	
−6	075	0.9	0.5	0630–0730
−5	094	2.8	1.4	0730–0830
−4	100	4.2	2.1	0830–0930
−3	100	4.6	2.3	0930–1030
−2	100	3.6	1.8	1030–1130
−1	095	1.8	0.9	1130–1230
HW	320	0.4	0.2	1230–1330

TIDAL STREAMS

The vertical rise and fall of the tide is the result of the horizontal movement of water known as a *tidal stream*. There are specific positions on a chart marked by a diamond shape enclosing a letter, called *tidal diamonds*. To one side of the chart there is a table which gives the true direction of the tidal flow together with its rate in knots (nautical miles per hour) for both spring and neap tides. This table is based on HW at the closest standard port and gives hourly intervals before and after. Tidal stream tabulations are based on mean (average) measurements so that tidal streams at spring tides are faster.

Tidal stream atlas

Fig 7.17 shows an extract from a tidal stream atlas giving Channel tide movements at HW Dover and six hours later. The arrows represent the direction of flow; you can see that at HW the flow is westwards and six hours later it is going in the opposite direction. The figures next to the arrows give the speed in knots for neaps and springs. Conventionally, the decimal point is omitted. So at HW off Land's End the flow is west–going at 0.8 knots for

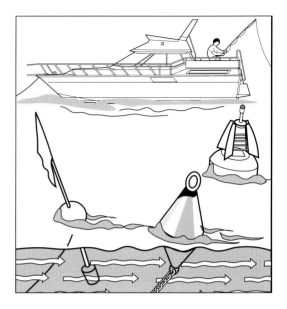

Fig 7.21   *You can check on the direction of the tidal stream by observing the pull on buoys, lobster pot markers and moored boats.*

neaps and 1.4 knots for springs (shown as 08,14).

Observing the tidal stream

There is normally no tidal stream information for areas close inshore. Sometimes information on local effects is given in sailing directions or pilot books. Generally a tidal stream does not flow as strongly in

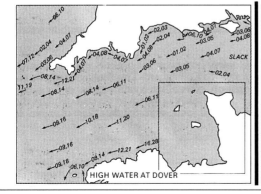
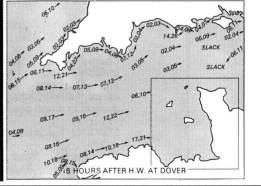

Fig 7.17   *Extract from a tidal stream atlas.*

shallow water; and in a bay it may sweep round in a contrary direction to the main stream. However it tends to flow faster around headlands sometimes causing severe tide races or overfalls where the water is very confused: see Fig 7.18 showing overfalls off St Catherine's Point. It can also well up from an uneven bottom causing disturbed seas and eddies. These areas should be avoided particularly if the wind is blowing in the opposite direction to the tidal stream.

Take every opportunity to observe the direction and rate of the tidal stream on passing moored boats, buoys and lobster pot markers, Fig 7.21. In a river or tidal estuary the strongest current or tidal stream, and the deepest water, lie on the outside of a bend; the inside frequently silts up. If there are no buoys, beacons or withies (markers), do not cut the corners on bends. A tidal stream flowing over a shallow bank often produces a standing wave just downstream of the bank so watch out for these.

QUESTIONS

7.1   What is chart datum?

7.2   Can the tide ever fall below chart datum?

7.3   a)   What is charted depth?
      b)   How is this shown on a chart.

7.4   What datum level is used when indicating the height of land features?

7.5   When does the greatest range of tide occur?

7.6   Where can information be obtained on times and heights of tides?

7.7   A boat with a draught of 2.0 m needs a clearance of 0.5 m to cross a sandbar which dries 1.3 m. What is the height of tide required?

7.8   What is the height of tide at Dover on 17 June at 1920 BST (Figs 7.5 and 7.6)?

7.9   At what time (BST) during the afternoon of 1 June will the tide first rise to a height of 2.5 m at Ramsgate (Figs 7.5, 7.6 and 7.8)?

7.10 What is the height of tide at Yarmouth at 1015 BST on 2 June (Figs 7.12, 7.13 and 7.14)?

7.11 What is the direction and rate of the tidal stream at spring tides one hour after high water in position at tidal diamond K (Fig 7.18)?

7.12 See 6.8. The tidal stream at tidal diamond B is 026° 03 kn. The wind is from the west. The boats at anchor in Studland Bay have their bows pointing to the west. Why?

7.13 Approaching the Needles Fairway buoy (to the west of the Isle of Wight), how can you check on the direction of the tidal stream?

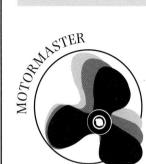

CHAPTER EIGHT

PRINCIPLES OF PILOTAGE

FINDING YOUR WAY BY LAND-MARKS AND SEAMARKS

To begin with, you will be making short passages relatively close to the shore in good visibility. Under these conditions you can rely on what you can see to establish your position and to work out the direction to go. There are many landmarks such as headlands, lighthouses, churches, and water towers; there are also buoys and beacons (see Chapter 9 Buoyage). Using a chart to identify these marks, they become signposts to establish the boat's present position and where to go next; this is **pilotage**. Should the visibility deteriorate and the signposts disappear, then it will be necessary to start plotting on the chart; and pilotage becomes navigation.

Pilotage is all about finding your way safely at sea. In this unfamiliar, ever changing environment, everything around takes on a new meaning. Distance becomes difficult to estimate, especially when it is dark. All around there are unseen underwater hazards waiting for the unwary. There are shingle banks to negotiate, patches of shallow water, rocks, places where the tidal stream speeds up and causes turbulence and many other problems.

At first glance the uninitiated may be completely bewildered and decide that this frightening experience is not for them, but forearmed with the correct information, all of these hazards can be avoided. Although there are no written signs, there are signposts such as buoys, marks on the shore and lights at night. Even the depth of water can be found simply by measuring with a weight on a line. However, by themselves these things are of little value in an unfamiliar area. When the boat is alongside a floating mark, it is necessary to know what it is, what it means, where it is and where to go from it to the next mark. It is also necessary to know if there are any hazards along the proposed track (course). Knowing the depth of water under the boat is fine when anchoring but, when underway, it is necessary to know depths of water ahead and to each side of the boat.

A plan is essential for accurate pilotage. Once you have checked the chart and pilot book (see Chapter 13) note down your passage plan in a *pilotage notebook*.

The plan gives sufficient information so that the chart and pilot need only be consulted should doubt over a detail arise.

Often the safe track which the boat must follow does not allow for any but minor deviations. Therefore, should an unexpected alteration of course be unavoidable, you must know the presence of hazards either side of the track.

ROCKS

Chart symbols for dangerous rocks are shown here together with a profile which gives you an idea of how they would look under water.

1 Rock (yellow on chart) which does not cover. The figure shown is the height above mean high water springs (MHWS).

2 This indicates a rock which covers and uncovers. The height above chart datum is given if known. The underlined figure indicates the drying height ie the rock is 3.5 metres *above* the level of chart datum.

3 A star (which could have a dotted circle round it) shows a small rock which, like **2** covers and uncovers.

4. A cross with dots in its angles shows a rock which is awash at chart datum level.

5 A cross without dots shows a rock of which the depth is unknown but could be a danger.

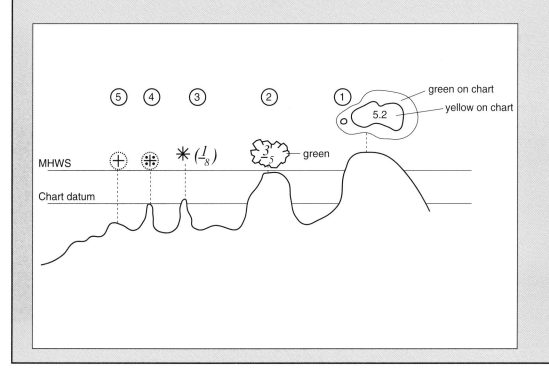

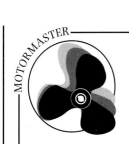
RIVER RUNS

Most of the dangers that you will face will probably be on the approaches to harbour. This is why it is unwise to attempt to leave or enter a harbour until you have carefully studied a large-scale chart of the area.

Small river navigation can present particular hazards. For example if you wish to visit Christchurch harbour in Dorset you have to negotiate the river Stour past Mudeford Quay. The navigable channel is very narrow as there is a shingle bank and sand bar which tend to shift after winter storms, altering the depths in the channel. Although it is buoyed in summer, it is still tricky because you have to avoid wind surfers and dinghies tacking to and fro. The Run past the quay averages 3 to 5 knots with the outgoing stream even reaching 9 knots. A small motor cruiser may have a bit of a struggle against this stream plus you have the benefit of a large fascinated audience of holiday makers in summer, so make sure that you check your tide tables (see Chapter 7).

The photograph shows the approximate course you would take to approach The Run by Mudeford Quay from the south, being very careful to follow the buoyed channel as it is all too easy to run aground on the sand bank. Here you can also see one of the local very fast-moving hazards: windsurfers.

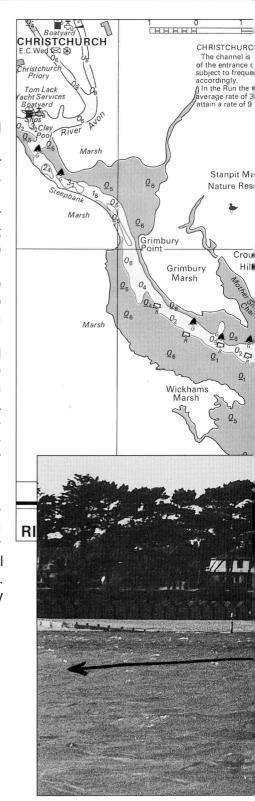

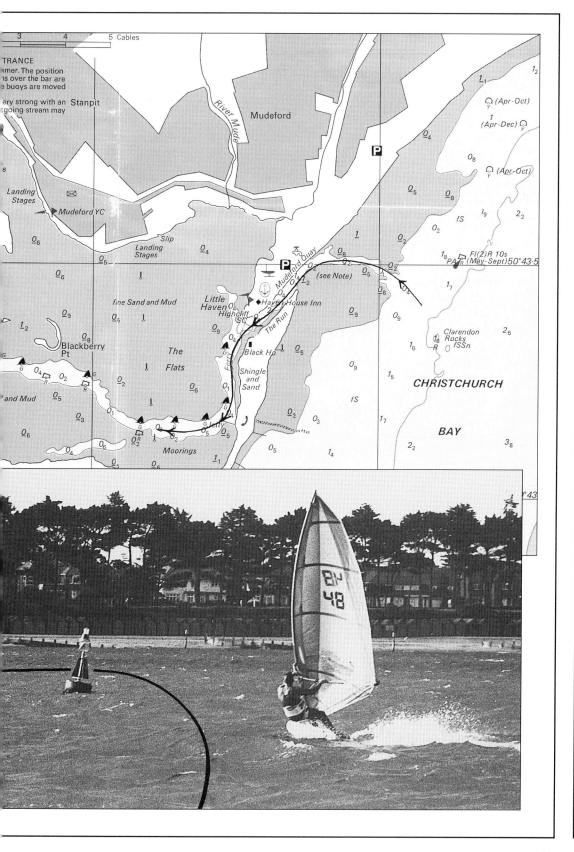

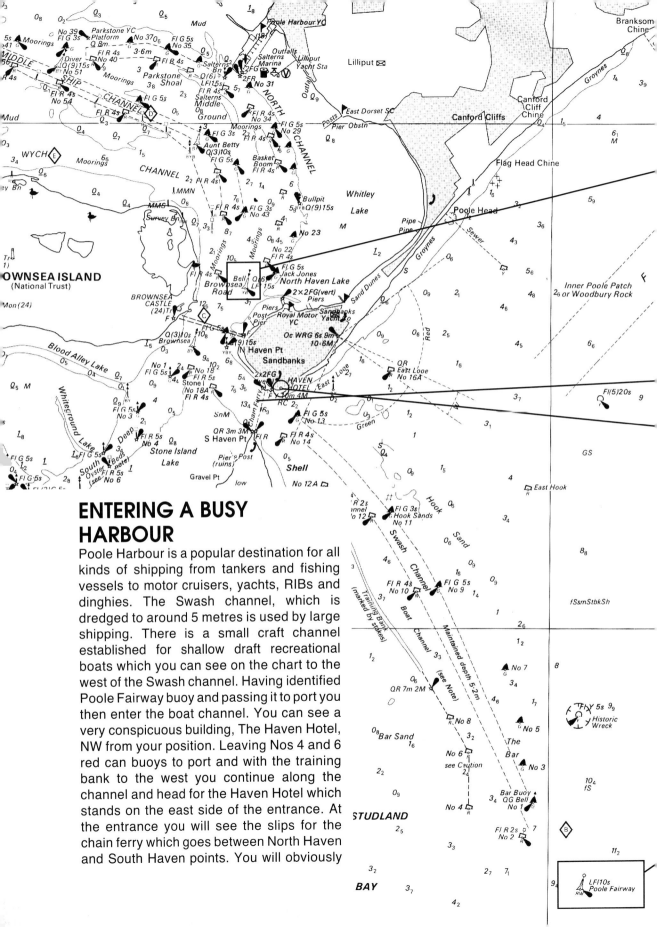

ENTERING A BUSY HARBOUR

Poole Harbour is a popular destination for all kinds of shipping from tankers and fishing vessels to motor cruisers, yachts, RIBs and dinghies. The Swash channel, which is dredged to around 5 metres is used by large shipping. There is a small craft channel established for shallow draft recreational boats which you can see on the chart to the west of the Swash channel. Having identified Poole Fairway buoy and passing it to port you then enter the boat channel. You can see a very conspicuous building, The Haven Hotel, NW from your position. Leaving Nos 4 and 6 red can buoys to port and with the training bank to the west you continue along the channel and head for the Haven Hotel which stands on the east side of the entrance. At the entrance you will see the slips for the chain ferry which goes between North Haven and South Haven points. You will obviously

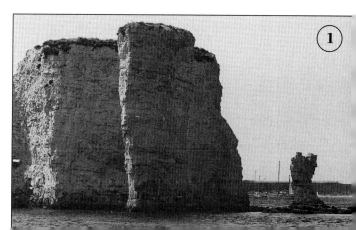

have to keep well clear of this vessel but, as you are under power, there should not be a problem. Beyond the entrance you will see Brownsea Island and Castle. The next seamark to look for is the Bell buoy at Brownsea Road which marks the division between the North channel and the Middle Ship channel, which you will take, branching west to Poole Town Quay.

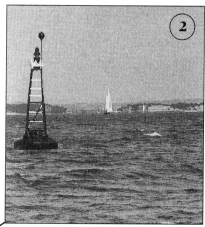

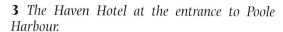

5 *The south cardinal Bell buoy at Brownsea Road which marks the division between the North and Middle ship channels.*

4 *The chain ferry at North Haven Point. Notice the prominent black ball forward which shows direction of travel.*

3 *The Haven Hotel at the entrance to Poole Harbour.*

2 *Once in Studland Bay, look out for Poole Fairway red and white safe water buoy which marks the Poole approach. The training bank is visible to port and the conspicuous Haven Hotel can be seen in the distance.*

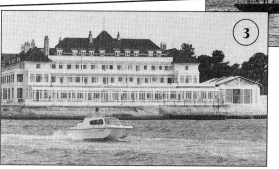

1 *Approaching from the southwest you will pass Handfast Point with the very recognisable Old Harry Rock.*

Starting at the bottom of this page you can follow the approach to Poole Harbour through a series of photographs linked to their position on the chart.

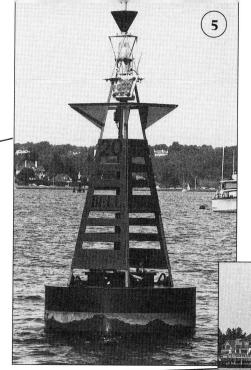

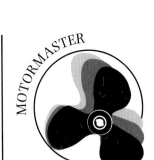

CHAPTER NINE

BUOYAGE

IALA BUOYAGE SYSTEM

The International Association of Lighthouse Authorities (IALA) is made up of representatives from countries all over the world and it is responsible for the formulation of worldwide buoyage systems. Each country is responsible for erecting and maintaining its own navigational aids.

In the United Kingdom, Trinity House, London, is the sole authority for providing lights and is responsible for fixed and floating seamarks. Although some local authorities maintain seamarks within their own port limits these are inspected regularly by Trinity House and any changes must first be sanctioned by them.

In the United States of America, the US Coastguard is responsible for all lights and other navigational aids along the US coastline and its possessions. There are also some private aids to navigation maintained by individuals.

Conventional direction of buoyage

The conventional direction of buoyage can be recognised in two ways:

- The direction taken on the approach to a harbour, estuary or river from seaward.

- A clockwise direction round large land masses.

Buoys are plentiful in the approaches to commercial ports. For smaller harbours and

Cardinal buoys indicate the direction of danger. Above right: an east cardinal buoy. Right: a north cardinal buoy.

secondary channels, beacons are used extensively. Occasionally, down infrequently used channels, tree branches (called *withies*) are stuck in the mud to indicate the limits of the deep water.

For an unfamiliar passage, where a buoyed channel is to be followed, it is a good idea to

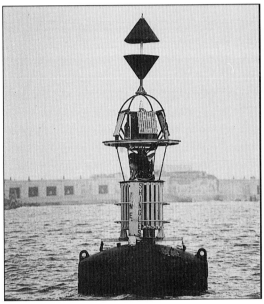

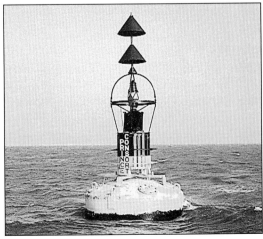

MOTORMASTER

draw up a list of the buoys (or beacons) to help identify them. Sufficient characteristics should be included so that it will not be necessary to keep returning to the chart table to check. If there is any doubt about visibility, the direction and distance of the next mark (buoy or beacon) should be noted.

At night, particular attention needs to be paid to the light characteristics of those buoys and beacons that are lit. From low down in a boat it is very difficult to judge distances, so tick off the lights (on the list) as you identify them. A watch with a second hand (or a digital stop watch) is useful for checking the characteristics of lights. Remember, too, that lights on buoys are not often visible at distances greater than two nautical miles. If the colour of a light is not indicated it is assumed to be white.

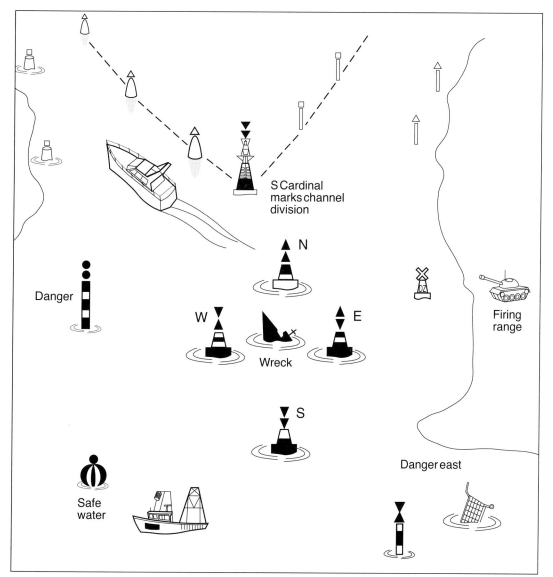

Fig 9.1 *This scene gives an idea of how buoyage is used.*

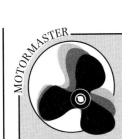
TYPES OF MARKS

There are five types of mark used. These are distinguished during the day by colour, shape and topmark; though sometimes the colour may not be very obvious due to weathering. During the night they can be identified by a light showing a distinctive colour and rhythm. Some marks have sound signals for their location in poor visibility. See inside the front cover of this book for colour illustrations of buoys.

Lateral marks

These indicate the lateral limits of a navigable channel. When proceeding in the general direction of buoyage, for IALA System A used in the UK, Europe and Africa, red marks will be left to port and green marks to starboard. (For IALA System B used in North and South America, red marks will be left to starboard and green marks to port.)

Lateral marks show defined channels.

The port markers are can-shaped or show a can shape on top and may have a red flashing light. These should always be to your left when approaching from seaward. To help tell which is which remember, that port wine is red. Starboard marks are cone-shaped and may have a green flashing light. They should always be to your right when approaching from seaward.

Safe water marks

A safe water mark indicates safe water all around it. It is used as a mid-channel or fairway mark or to indicate landfall (first sight of land).

These marks have red and white

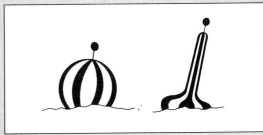

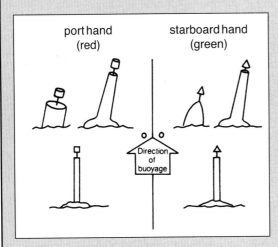

port hand
(red)

starboard hand
(green)

Direction
of
buoyage

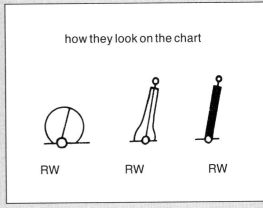

how they look on the chart

RW   RW   RW

vertical stripes and may appear as a sphere, a pillar or a spar. If a light is fitted, it will be white: isophase, occulting or Morse A (see Fig 10.1).

Cardinal marks

Cardinal marks are based on four points of the compass. Their job is to indicate the limits of hazards. Each mark has its own code of top-mark, colour and light characteristic.

The colours are yellow and black in various sequences. You will need to memorise the shapes: **N**orth and **S**outh are easy as they have double 'arrows' pointing up and down. **E**ast looks a bit **E**gg shaped and **W**est looks like a **W**ine glass. See the coloured end paper for the light sequences.

Isolated danger

Isolated danger marks are buoyed over the danger with safe water at a distance around the buoy. They are coloured red and black with 2 spheres as a top mark. If there is a light it is white, group flashing (2).

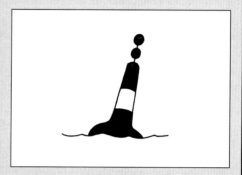

Special marks (non-navigational)

A special mark is a non-navigational mark used to show a special feature which may be shown on the chart. They could indicate a spoil ground, military exercise zones (marked DZ), or sewer outfall. The shapes vary but the colour is always yellow with an X shape on top.

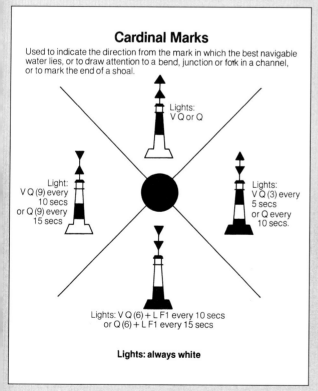

Cardinal Marks

Used to indicate the direction from the mark in which the best navigable water lies, or to draw attention to a bend, junction or fork in a channel, or to mark the end of a shoal.

Lights:
V Q or Q

Light:
V Q (9) every
10 secs
or Q (9) every
15 secs

Lights:
V Q (3) every
5 secs
or Q every
10 secs.

Lights: V Q (6) + L Fl every 10 secs
or Q (6) + L Fl every 15 secs

Lights: always white

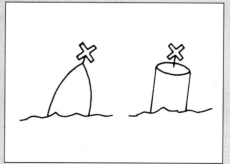

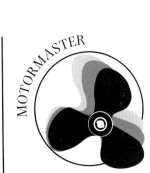

LIGHTS, LIGHTHOUSES & PORT TRAFFIC SIGNALS

Your first few passages will probably be made in daylight. Nevertheless, you should still learn a little about lights – in case your journey takes longer than expected and you reach harbour after dark. Lights and signals in poor visibility are dealt with in Chapter 23, in the section on safety at sea.

Lights used for navigational purposes are marked on the chart with a magenta blob. Lights may be in lighthouses or in the windows of buildings, and are on some buoys and beacons.

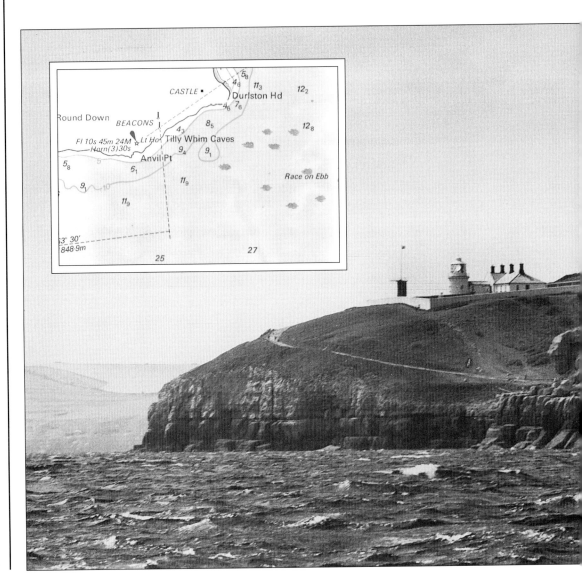

LIGHT CHARACTERISTICS

So that you can identify lights easily they have different characteristics which are shown in Fig 10.1.

Anvil Point lighthouse. The insert shows a section of a chart giving the lighthouse's location and light characteristics. The abbreviations next to the light show that it flashes every 10 seconds; it is 45 metres above the highest water level (mean high water springs); in good weather it has a nominal range of 24 miles. It also has a fog signal which emits 3 blasts every 30 seconds.

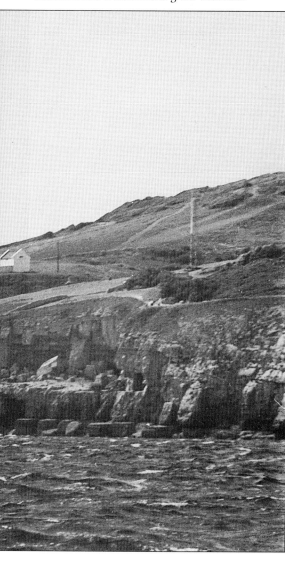

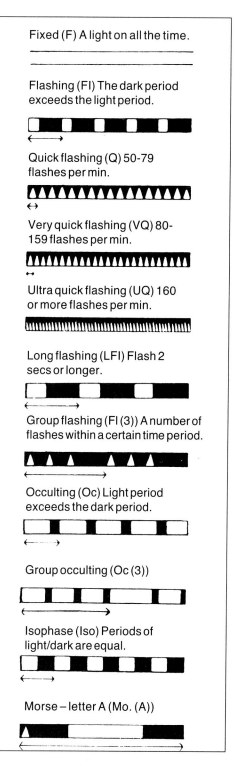

Fixed (F) A light on all the time.

Flashing (Fl) The dark period exceeds the light period.

Quick flashing (Q) 50-79 flashes per min.

Very quick flashing (VQ) 80-159 flashes per min.

Ultra quick flashing (UQ) 160 or more flashes per min.

Long flashing (LFl) Flash 2 secs or longer.

Group flashing (Fl (3)) A number of flashes within a certain time period.

Occulting (Oc) Light period exceeds the dark period.

Group occulting (Oc (3))

Isophase (Iso) Periods of light/dark are equal.

Morse – letter A (Mo. (A))

Fig 10.1 *Key to identification of lights on buoys and beacons.*

MOTORMASTER

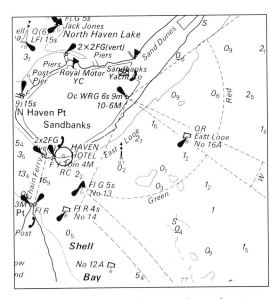

Fig 10.2 *An extract from a chart showing a sectored light. You know that you are on the right approach when you can only see the white sector.*

Lights may have coloured sectors (white, green and red) which can show navigational hazards or tell you where a channel is. If you look at Fig 10.2 you can see a light to the right of the Haven Hotel. The abbreviations next to the light show us that it is an occulting single light (showing more light than dark) sectored white, red and green flashing every 6 seconds; its height is 9 metres above mean high water springs and the lights are visible for 10 miles (white) and 6 miles (red and green). The straight dotted lines coming from it show the white sector marking the East Looe channel into Poole Harbour. To the right and left of the white sector are red

Fig 10.3 *Corbière lighthouse on Jersey warns mariners of the treacherous reefs below it. Notice the other landmarks: a tower and chimney.*

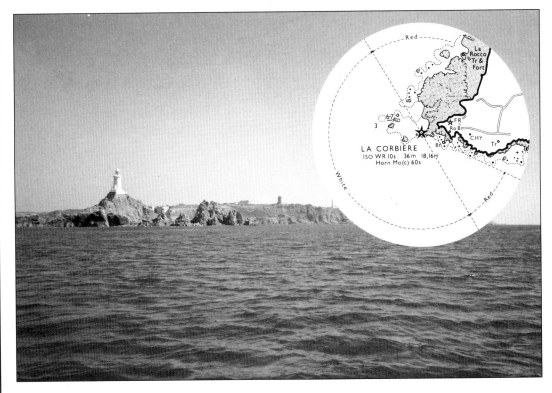

LEADING MARKS AND LIGHTS

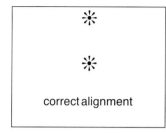

correct alignment

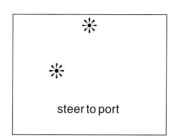

steer to port

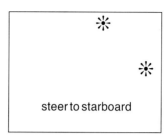

steer to starboard

A very useful set of aids to entering or leaving an unfamiliar harbour is a set of leading marks or lights. Once you have lined up the pair correctly you then know that you are heading into the safe water channel.

Looking at Fig 10.4 you can see that the leading lights are identified on the chart extract by Ldg F R 7,5m 4M (leading lights fixed red with heights of 7 and 5 metres, visible 4 miles out to sea). The tricky thing is identifying the correct pair amongst all the other lights visible in a busy harbour.

However you are also given a compass bearing of 244° magnetic so that you can confirm that you are focussed on the correct pair of lights. The chart or almanac will give you other information to help you find the safe approach.

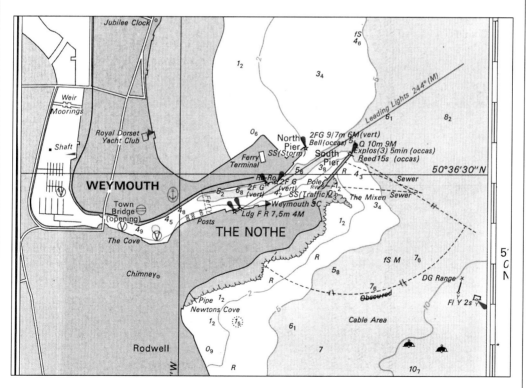

Fig 10.4 *Leading lights on Weymouth harbour to show the way in by a safe channel.*

and green sectors; as you approach if you stray to starboard you will see a red light and to port you will see a green light. If you are properly on course you will only see white. If you look the light up in an almanac it will tell you the angles of the sectors; in this case they are: red 234°–294°; white 294°–304°; green 304°–024°. These bearings are given as they are seen from seaward.

DIPPING LIGHTS (CALCULATING THE DISTANCE OFF A LIGHTHOUSE)

Looking at the chart extract showing Anvil Point lighthouse on page 66, you may wonder why the height of the lighthouse is given. It is because a simple way of estimating the distance away from it or 'distance off' has been worked out. The curvature of the earth limits the range at which the

The East Looe can buoy shown on the chart extract on page 68. You will see this as you approach Poole Harbour from the east and need to round it closely to port to avoid sandbanks.

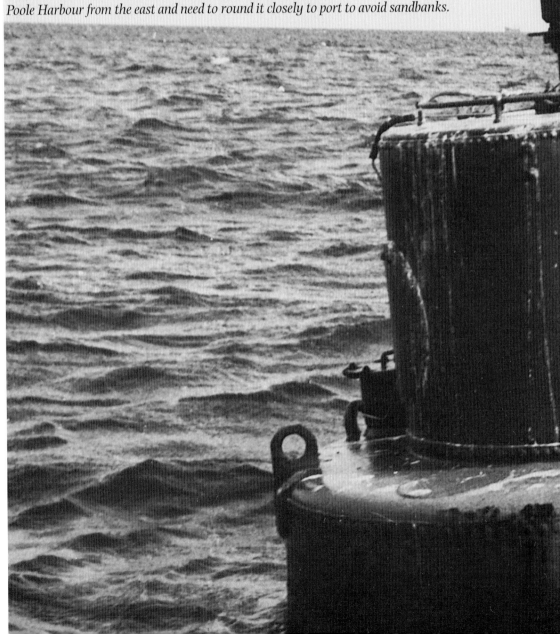

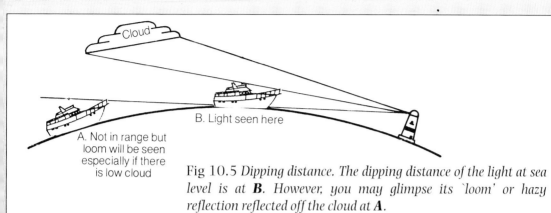

Fig 10.5 *Dipping distance. The dipping distance of the light at sea level is at* **B**. *However, you may glimpse its 'loom' or hazy reflection reflected off the cloud at* **A**.

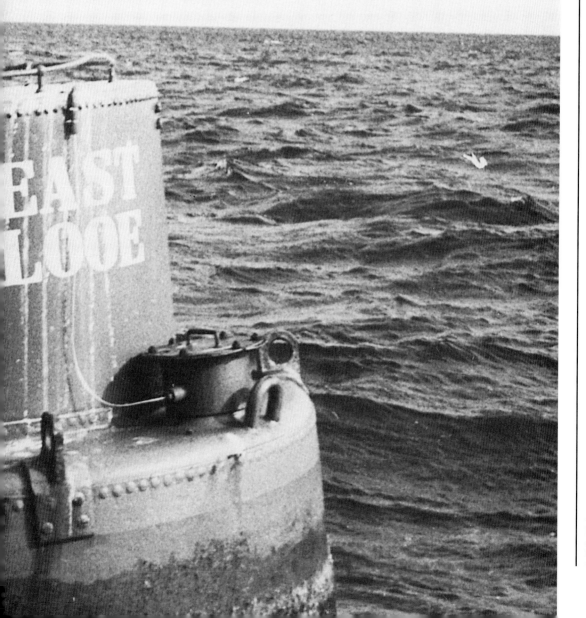

Height of Light		HEIGHT OF EYE						
		Metres						
		1.5	3	4.6	6.1	7.6	9.1	10.7
		Feet						
		5	10	15	20	25	30	35
m	ft							
12	40	9¾	11	11¾	12½	13	13½	14
15	50	10¾	11¾	12½	13¼	14	14½	15
18	60	11½	12½	13½	14	14¾	15¼	15¾
21	70	12¼	13¼	14	14¾	15½	16	16½
24	80	13	14	14¾	15½	16	16½	17
27	90	13½	14½	15½	16	16¾	17¼	17¾
30	100	14	15	16	16½	17¼	17¾	18¼
34	110	14½	15¾	16½	17¼	17¾	18¼	19
37	120	15¼	16¼	17	17¾	18¼	19	19½
40	130	15¾	16¾	17½	18¼	19	19½	20
43	140	16¼	17¼	18	18¾	19½	20	20½
46	150	16¾	17¾	18½	19¼	19¾	20½	21
49	160	17	18¼	19	19¾	20¼	20¾	21½
52	170	17½	18½	19½	20	20¾	21¼	21¾
55	180	18	19	20	20½	21¼	21¾	22¼
58	190	18½	19½	20¼	21	21½	22	22¾
61	200	18¾	20	20¾	21½	22	22½	23
64	210	19¼	20¼	21	21¾	22½	23	23½
67	220	19½	20¾	21½	22¼	22¾	23¼	24
70	230	20	21	22	22½	23¼	23¾	24¼
73	240	20½	21½	22¼	23	23½	24	24½
76	250	20¾	21¾	22½	23¼	24	24½	25
79	260	21	22¼	23	23¾	24¼	24¾	25¼
82	270	21½	22½	23¼	24	24½	25¼	25¾
85	280	21¾	23	23¾	24½	25	25½	26
88	290	22	23¼	24	24¾	25¼	26	26½
91	300	22½	23½	24½	25	25¾	26¼	26¾
95	310	22¾	24	24¾	25½	26	26½	27
98	320	23	24¼	25	25¾	26¼	27	27½
100	330	23½	24½	25¼	26	26½	27¼	27¾
104	340	23¾	24¾	25¾	26¼	27	27½	28
107	350	24	25	26	26¾	27¼	27¾	28¼
122	400	25½	26½	27½	28	28¾	29¼	29¾
137	450	27	28	28¾	29½	30	30¾	31¼

Fig 10.6 *Extract from a table in an almanac to give the distance of lights rising or dipping.*

light can be seen. This actually helps us because, due to the uniformity of the curve, we can work out how far away the light is from the point when it comes into view (see Fig 10.5). If you know the height of the light and your own height of eye above sea level you can look at a table in your nautical almanac which will tell you how many nautical miles the light is from your position when you first see the light. This is sometimes known as the rising or dipping distance because when motoring towards or away from a lighthouse at night a point is reached when the light appears to 'rise' or 'dip' above and below the horizon. Obviously to use this distance measurement you have to be able to identify correctly which light you have sighted.

As an example, look at the table in Fig 10.6. Assuming that your height of eye above water level is about 3 metres and taking the light height as 46 metres you will see that when the light rises into your vision you will then be approximately 17¾ miles from the lighthouse.

The higher you are above sea level, the greater the distance the light will be visible. If you take a compass bearing of the light at the same time you can get a fix of your position (see next chapter).

You must be sure that it is the real light you are looking at. It could be a reflection off a cloud giving a hazy image called a 'loom'.

PORT TRAFFIC SIGNALS

In a busy harbour, especially one which has commercial shipping there will probably be traffic control signals. Your pilot book or almanac will tell you what to look out for.

International Port Traffic Signals

Many commercial ports use the International Port Traffic Signals which are shown in Fig 10.7. These signals must be obeyed, even by small motor cruisers. Check in your pilot book for the correct VHF channel for Harbour Traffic Control and call in to seek instructions.

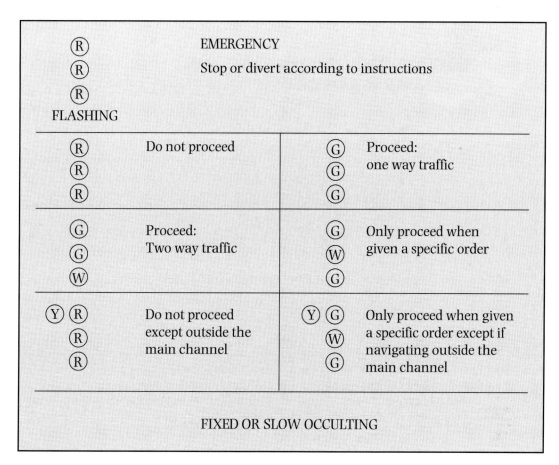

Fig 10.7 *International Port Traffic Signals.*

QUESTIONS
(Chapters 9 and 10)

9.1   You are on a northerly course and you sight ahead of you the buoy shown in the top photo on page 62. On which side should you pass it?

9.2   You see a white light VQ (9) 10s.
a)   What is it?
b)   Where is the hazard?

9.3   You are making a night approach to the East Looe channel, (chart extract page 68). Between what bearings would you expect to see the white sector of the East Looe Light Beacon (Oc WRG 6s)?

10.1   You are approaching an unfamiliar harbour when you see displayed at the entrance three flashing red lights in a vertical line.
a)   What do these lights signify?
b)   What should you do?

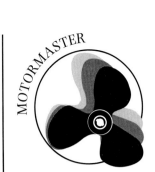

CHAPTER ELEVEN

TRANSITS AND CLEARING BEARINGS

Provided you know your approximate position on the chart (see Chapter 14), you can work out the magnetic bearing of a landmark or seamark that you are looking for. Then you use a hand-bearing compass to check your direction and identify the land/seamark. You have to be careful not to assume that the white building you spot is the conspicuous hotel marked on the chart – it may be a recently-built block of flats in an entirely different location. This is where your chartwork comes in; if you have been careful about plotting your position throughout your passage you won't make this kind of mistake.

TRANSITS

The extension of a line joining two fixed objects is known as a transit. (see Fig 11.1). It is the same principle as lining up

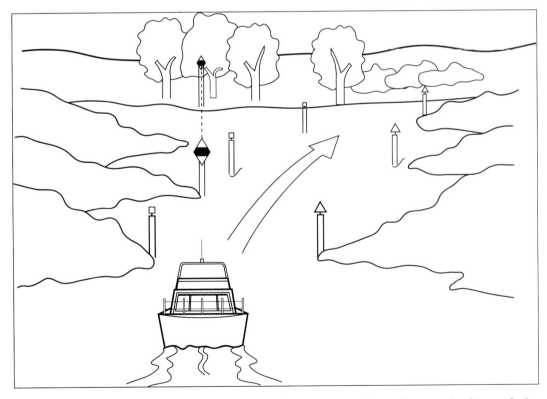

Fig 11.1 *Transit marks. As the boat approaches the river mouth you line up the diamonds for the entrance then keep within the port and starboard marks upriver. Sometimes the marks may only be sticks (withies) pushed into the soft mud.*

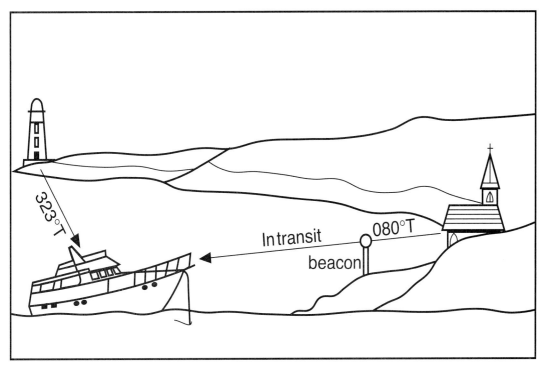

Fig 11.2 *Using transits with a bearing to find a safe anchorage marked on a chart. The boat drops anchor when the beacon and the church are in transit and the lighthouse bears 323°T.*

leading lights (see page Fig 10.4). You can tell when you are off–line to port or starboard when the two marks or beacons go out of alignment.

In open water you can use a transit to check your progress against a strong crossing tidal stream by lining up a buoy with a fixed point on the coastline.

A transit used with a compass bearing will give a good fix of position – useful for situations such as locating an anchorage (see Fig 11.2). When approaching a secluded anchorage in a small bay there may be a cross wind or cross tidal stream. Having established the boat's position in the approach to the anchorage and worked out where to anchor, then any two objects on the shore directly beyond the anchorage position can be kept in line on the approach. Once anchored, a further transit at right angles to the original transit can be established so that

the two can be used as a visual check that the boat is not dragging her anchor.

Transits can also be used to determine the moment to alter course. On a reasonably steep coastline, the left and right hard edges of the cliffs can be used as a transit (Fig 11.3).

BACK BEARINGS

Once you head away from the anchorage you can use the bearing of the object (in this case the church) to find your way out through rocks or sand bars to clear water by getting a member of the crew to look back at the church using the hand-bearing compass on the correct bearing. He or she can then tell you if you are veering off to port or starboard.

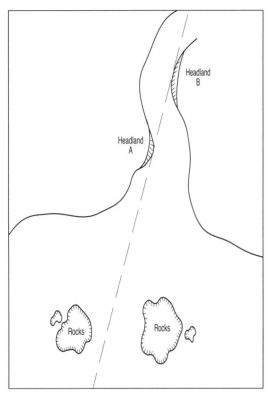

Fig 11.3 *Use of a steep coastline as a transit. The right-hand edge of the cliff at A is in transit with the left-hand edge of the cliff at B for a safe approach into the river.*

CLEARING BEARINGS

Underwater hazards and shallows will be shown on a chart but there may not always be a buoy to mark them. One way of avoiding dangers is to draw a clearing

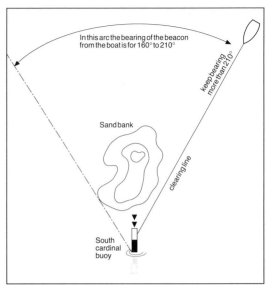

Fig 11.4 *A clearing bearing. Mark a clearing line on the chart using a known buoy or beacon to guide yourself through safe water. Here a south cardinal buoy marks a sandbank; a clearing line with a reciprocal bearing of 210°M has been determined. As you head towards the hazard if you keep your heading more than 210°M you will be in safe water.*

line *from* a charted buoy or beacon on the chart (a reciprocal bearing) to pass clear of the danger. Once you have measured the direction of this line, known as a *clearing bearing* you will then know that, provided you don't cross the clearing line, you will stay in safe water (see Fig 11.4).

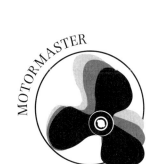

CHAPTER TWELVE

PILOTAGE SKILLS

LEAVING HARBOUR

Pilotage starts as soon as the boat leaves the berth. If you are familiar with the harbour and river there is no problem. In harbours where there are adequate marks and no offlying dangers it is simply a case of following the marks. When there are complications in an unfamiliar harbour, more research and action should be taken:

• Obtain a local plan of the harbour from the harbour master or marina manager, together with other relevant information. Yacht clubs may also have useful information.

• A large scale harbour chart should be available upon which to mark key points for quick reference, or a plan can be drawn in your pilotage notebook.

• Study your pilot book and almanac and jot down important details in your pilotage notebook.

• Keep checking your echo sounder for depth soon after leaving the berth and at any point along the way, until relatively deep water is reached.

• Check your tide tables. A strong tidal stream setting across the entrance of the harbour or river may make pilotage at slower speeds difficult if not impossible, especially if there is also a strong wind.

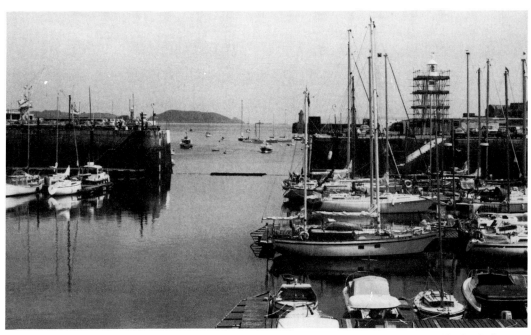

The marina in Victoria Basin, St Peter Port, Guernsey. Across the marina is a sill which dries at low tide so you can only leave harbour 2½ hours either side of HW, earlier if you have a deep draught or it is neap tides.

- Listen to the weather forecast. Strong winds from a given direction for a particular location may make it difficult to leave the berth or to pass safely through the harbour entrance especially if it is narrow. It may not be possible to see vital transits or clearing bearings in poor visibility.

- In commercial harbours and rivers, check whether permission is required before departure or before using any busy stretch of the river.

- Listen to the Port Radio Traffic on VHF radio.

- Find out well beforehand what harbour signals are displayed, particularly controlling entrance and exit and indicating water depth (see end of Chapter 10).

- Write down any transits or clearing bearings needed to avoid offlying dangers (see Chapter 11).

CRUISING ALONG THE COAST

Again, you should prepare information for a safe passage plan beforehand. (See Chapter 26 Coastal Passage Plan: Poole to Christchurch).

- Plot the required track or tracks on the chart seeing that any offlying dangers are cleared (see Chapter 14).

- Plot any clearing bearings and transits with the expected time of arrival at these points. If conditions make it impossible to use a hand-bearing compass, write down the time when these features should be abeam.

- Check that there is sufficient depth of water along your track at low water.

- Look at the chart to see whether there is a convenient depth contour line parallel to the shore which can be safely followed using the echo sounder.

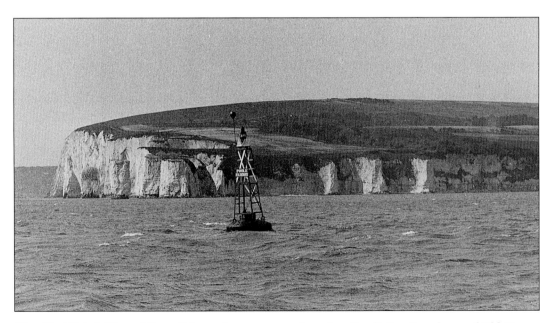

Handfast Point. Viewed from this angle, even on a clear day the distinctive shape of Old Harry Rock is indistinguishable from the headland. Here at least you have a buoy to fix your position.

MOTORMASTER

- List any hazards near the track together with the maximum amount that the course could be altered to clear them safely.

When relatively close inshore in good visibility, it is possible to buoy-hop or use land features for pilotage. In some instances it is a good idea to make a diversion to seek out a buoy to find an accurate position first (see Fig 12.1). Headlands show up particularly well and should be used in preference to landmarks such as buildings which may be difficult to identify.

Plot your course on the chart as you go along between marks, then if visibility deteriorates you will know the direction to the next mark. Even in good visibility it is useful to know the approximate position of the next mark so that you avoid wrong identification.

Once underway, you should observe the direction and rate of the tidal stream by looking at moored boats, fishing floats and buoys. There may be little or no tabulated information available for areas close inshore. In bays, the tidal stream is generally weaker and sometimes in a contrary direction to the main flow, whereas around a headland it speeds up causing disturbed water (Fig 12.2).

Tidal streams do not noticeably affect

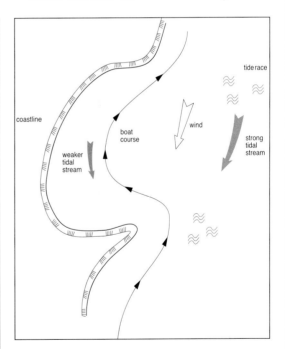

Fig 12.1 *It sometimes pays to divert into a bay where there is a known mark. It may take you a little longer but at least you are then confident that you know exactly where you are.*

Fig 12.2 *In this example you might think it would be better to cut across the bay from headland to headland. However, seeing that both wind and tide are against you, you would be better off diverting into the bay to motor round where the tidal stream is weaker and it is more sheltered from the wind. You will need to carefully check the chart for rocks and sand bars which may be potential hazards.*

BE CAUTIOUS WHEN USING PILOTAGE AIDS

Never assume that a headland that you have just sighted is the expected one. It is very easy to make it fit and draw the wrong conclusions. Look for distinguishing features to help identification.

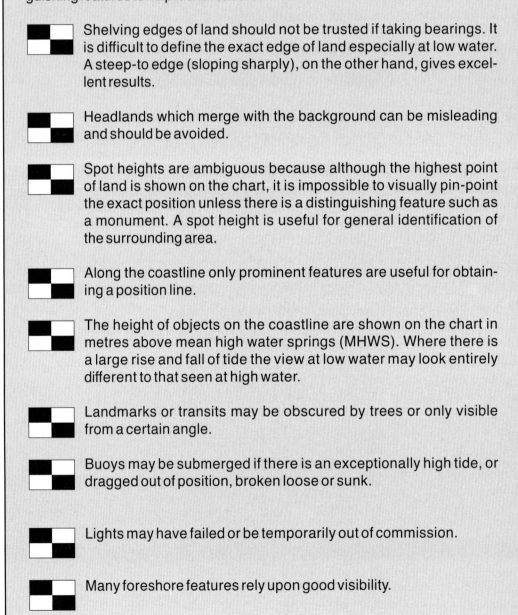

Shelving edges of land should not be trusted if taking bearings. It is difficult to define the exact edge of land especially at low water. A steep-to edge (sloping sharply), on the other hand, gives excellent results.

Headlands which merge with the background can be misleading and should be avoided.

Spot heights are ambiguous because although the highest point of land is shown on the chart, it is impossible to visually pin-point the exact position unless there is a distinguishing feature such as a monument. A spot height is useful for general identification of the surrounding area.

Along the coastline only prominent features are useful for obtaining a position line.

The height of objects on the coastline are shown on the chart in metres above mean high water springs (MHWS). Where there is a large rise and fall of tide the view at low water may look entirely different to that seen at high water.

Landmarks or transits may be obscured by trees or only visible from a certain angle.

Buoys may be submerged if there is an exceptionally high tide, or dragged out of position, broken loose or sunk.

Lights may have failed or be temporarily out of commission.

Many foreshore features rely upon good visibility.

motorboats travelling at high speeds and so a pre- determined track can safely be followed, but should the speed need to be reduced due to traffic density, poor visibility, engine failure or rough seas, care still must be taken to see that the boat is not set on to hazards by a tidal stream. In such a situation, the position should be established and course altered to ensure that the boat is on a safe track. If necessary clearing bearings or transits should be used (Fig 11.3).

APPROACHING HARBOUR

As with the rest of the pilotage plan, the harbour entrance plan should be prepared in good time as it is all too easy to leave this until the last minute causing a frantic search through pilotage notes and charts. An alternative destination should also be planned well ahead of time in case, for some reason, the original destination cannot be reached.

It is best to plan the initial visit to an unfamiliar harbour during daylight hours in good visibility rather than to attempt this at night when distance is difficult to judge. Some buoys are unlit and become a hazard rather than a help. It is also important to establish the leading lights for an approach to an estuary or harbour.

Here are some points to help you to plan your approach:

- Have all transits and clearing bearings written down well beforehand.

- In bad visibility consider the viability of setting a course well uptide of the harbour entrance so that when land is sighted there will be no doubt which way to follow the coast and there will also be a fair tide (See box feature on pages 82-3.)

- Depths shown on the chart and in the pilot book may be incorrect if the area is not surveyed frequently, or if silting has occurred and the channel is not dredged regularly. For this reason all depths should be regarded as an indication only and a margin for error allowed for. Always check the depth in the channel with your echo sounder.

- Be aware of any harbour regulations or bye laws and watch for harbour entrance signals.

- Find out, by reference to charts and pilotage notes, on which side of a narrow channel the deeper water lies so that in an emergency, your course can be altered in that direction if local rules allow, but remember that in some harbours smaller vessels must keep to certain designated areas shown on the chart.

- Be aware of any tidal stream or weather limitations for a particular harbour so that if conditions are likely to prevent safe entry, an alternative destination can be used.

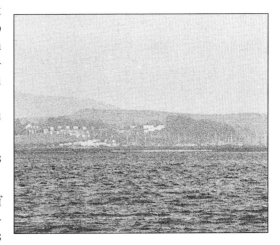

Wareham Lake. In hazy conditions, it may be hard to distinguish land or seamarks easily so you must plot your position in unfamiliar waters.

MOTORMASTER

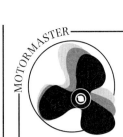

THE WRONG HEADLAND

When viewing an unfamiliar coastline, one bay looks very much like the next, headlands appear similar and it is easy to identify a feature incorrectly. Look for other clues. Perhaps there is a lighthouse on the headland or there are radio masts next to a church in a bay. Any such features can be used if they are marked on the chart or in the pilotage book.

It is, of course, easier to find a destination when land has been within sight the whole time than it is after a sea crossing out of sight of land. The following example shows how a problem of wrong identification could have been avoided.

A motorboat has just completed a Channel crossing and has sighted land. Visibility is good but it has been a rough passage and there has been some instrument failure. The navigator has not kept a record of the boat's estimated position and so is not certain where the boat is. Speed had to be reduced due to strong winds causing heavy seas. The initial course set was to the harbour entrance.

A headland with a lighthouse on it is sighted (see Fig 12.3) and it is assumed that this is Crab Point, so course is altered for the harbour entrance. Some time later the harbour has still not been sighted but another headland with a black banded lighthouse comes into view. Two aerials are seen to the left of the lighthouse. After consulting the chart the navigator realises that this is Crab Point and the other wrongly identified headland was Prawle Head. Due to reduced speed, the boat had been set (carried by the tidal stream) to the west of the harbour.

The tide is now ebbing and the stream is stronger and at reduced speed the boat is not making much headway. The harbour is eventually reached at low water. As the original plan had been to enter the harbour at high water the

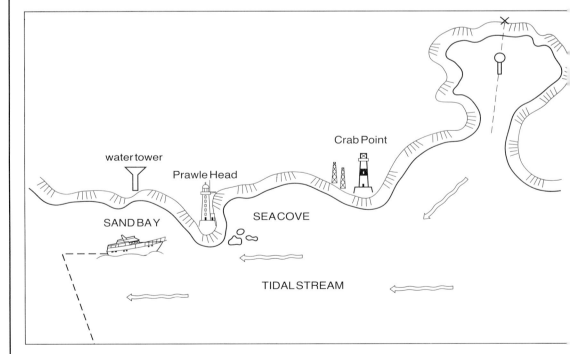

Fig 12.3 *It is often easy to mistake a headland.*

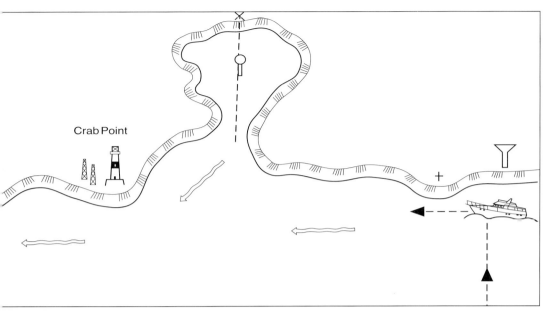

Fig 12.4 *A deliberate error uptide helps to locate the harbour entrance.*

navigator did not make a note of the leading marks which indicate the safe passage at low water. The boat misses the safe channel and goes aground, fortunately on soft mud and so no damage is done. As the tide is still falling there is a lengthy wait until the boat refloats.

Now let's see where things went wrong:

• A detailed plan should have been prepared which included the harbour entrance leading marks and identifying features along the coastline on either side of the harbour.

• If the chart and pilot had been consulted when land was sighted the navigator would have seen that the lighthouse on the headland did not have a black band and there were no aerials near to it, so it could not have been Crab Point. The only other lighthouse in the area was the one on Prawle Head. At this point the navigator should have looked along the coastline to see if there were any other identifying features such as the conspicuous water tower in Sand Bay. By using the lighthouse and the water tower the boat's position could have been established. Fortunately, visibility was

good and the navigator realised his error when Crab Point was sighted. In bad visibility, however, the error could have gone undiscovered which, when the headland was cleared and the course altered for the harbour entrance, could have caused the boat to ground on the rocks in Sea Cove.

• The estimated position (see page 101) should have been plotted at hourly intervals which would have shown that the boat was being set westwards.

• When speed was reduced, it would have been better to make a deliberate error uptide so that the tidal stream could have been used to advantage when land was sighted, (see Fig 12.4).

It is all too easy to rely upon instruments for position finding; these will do a very efficient job most of the time, but should they breakdown then other methods have to be used. Therefore, they should always be backed up with notes from the pilot book, tracks on the chart and personal observations. The boat's position should be plotted on the chart at regular intervals using any method available.

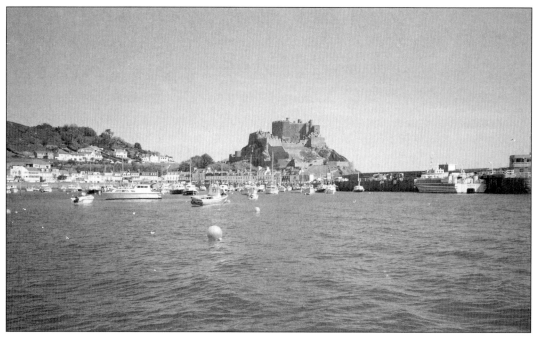

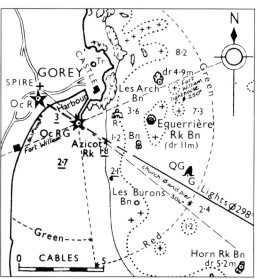

When approaching Gorey Harbour, Jersey, for the first time you have excellent conspicuous marks in the form of Mont Orgueil Castle, just north of the pier. As you can see from the chartlet (a typical presentation in a pilot book) there is also a church spire W of the castle. Gorey is a good example of a harbour where you need to do thorough homework as it dries out completely at low water.

- If the harbour operates on VHF radio then a call can be made on the appropriate channel. In the UK, a marina berth can be reserved by calling the marina on VHF channel 80.

- Find out whether there are any custom or immigration regulations in force and if so, the appropriate action to take.

- Consult the pilot book to see where the marinas are, and when and where fuel and water may be obtained.

- An inner harbour may only be accessible within a certain interval from high water so check on opening times and also where the boat can safely wait prior to entry.

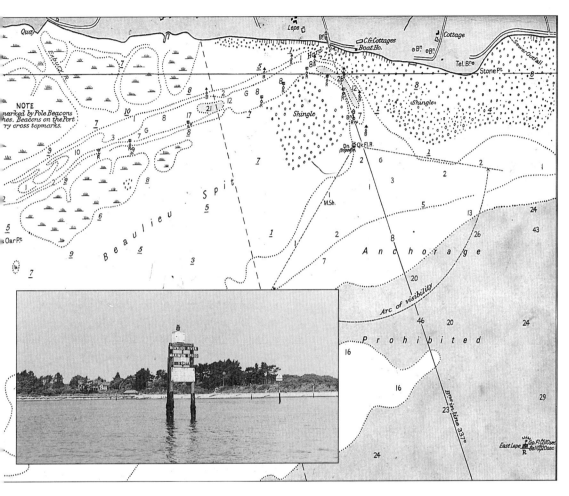

Fig 12.5 Charts of navigable rivers are obtainable giving essential information on the safe channels and depths (given here in feet). This extract from a chart of Beaulieu River, Hampshire, shows the entrance channel mark (see also inset) and the well-marked channel which threads its way through marshes. The chart tells us that the port hand beacons carry cross topmarks. Extract by courtesy of Imray Laurie, Norie & Wilson Ltd.

PILOTAGE INLAND

Those who never venture inland further than the first anchorage or marina miss a great deal. There are usually many unexpected surprises in store such as a quiet anchorage with a deserted beach, a small local restaurant, or a friendly little village.

It is sometimes easier to motor up river at low water, if there is sufficient depth, as then the channel can be clearly seen.

As with coastal pilotage, the pilot book and chart must be carefully studied and a plan made of what is ahead. With the close proximity of land and the plentiful supply of good landmarks, knowing the boat's position at any time is not a problem. However, there is usually a speed limit to be observed and in some areas, landing may be prohibited.

If the river flows directly into the sea the initial stretches will be tidal and the direction of the flow will reverse throughout the day in relation to the tidal stream for that area. This must be taken into consideration when anchoring, mooring or approaching a river bank. Additionally some areas may dry out.

Further upriver, although it will no longer be tidal, there may still be seasonal fluctuations in water level due to evaporation or heavy rainfall. The river current will no longer be affected by the tidal stream and so will always flow in the same direction.

In the lower reaches of a smaller river there will usually be small secondary buoys, beacons or posts but in the upper reaches there may be tree branches, known as withies, stuck in the mud either side of the channel, or no markings.

The rate at which the current flows may vary. In some areas where the current is strong it is better to keep to the shallow water near the bank when making way upstream and to take advantage of the faster flow towards the middle when proceeding downstream.

At a bend in the river, the deeper water is usually on the outer curve where the water is flowing faster. At the inner part of the bend where the flow is slower, silting occurs. Beware of obstructions jutting out from the river bank. Careful study of the chart in conjunction with visual observations will help you get a feel for river pilotage.

A general look at the topography of the area will help. If the bank is tree lined there will probably be roots sticking out from it; a steep sloping bank usually has deep water along it; whereas a gradually sloping bank may have a spit extending out into the river.

Canals

Canals offer access through quiet countryside. Originally intended for commercial traffic they are now mainly used for pleasure craft. Before venturing into a canal system study the appropriate canal guide for details of any local regulations and restrictions. Lock opening times, details of any dangers or canal closures should be obtained from the keeper at the first lock. Check to see that there is sufficient water along the entire system you propose to use, and consider the height and width of bridges to see that there is sufficient clearance. The boat should be well fendered especially when using the locks. Fenders are usually left secured in position when canal cruising. As with rivers there is a speed limit; excess speed in a canal can affect the boat's manoeuvrability.

The canal signs should be learned together with required sound signals. Canal guides will give details of mooring sites, shopping and toilet facilities, where fresh water is available, where fuel and gas can be obtained and where repair work can be done.

The canal may be very narrow and the water in some places too shallow near the banks, so boats should keep towards the middle. When another boat is approaching from ahead, both boats should move to their right and slow down. When the larger boat is parallel, the smaller boat should accelerate slightly to maintain steerage, otherwise it may be drawn towards the larger one.

Locks

Locks provide a method for boats to move from one level to a higher or lower level giving access to water which would otherwise be inaccessible. A lock consists of a

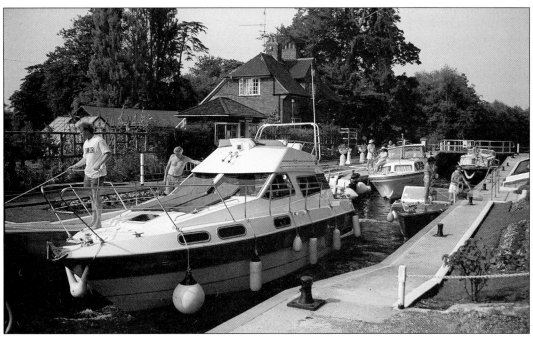

A crowded lock in summer. Boats are being secured by the passing of lines from stern and bow round bollards on the lock side. These can easily be slackened off as the water level lowers or in a filling lock, tightened as the level rises.

watertight basin with sluice gates at either end. When the gates are closed, the water level in the lock can be raised or lowered until it is the same level as the water on the outer side of one of the gates. This gate is opened and the boat proceeds along the canal to the next lock. Watch for pilotage signals when approaching a lock; these may vary from a complicated set of lights or shapes to the lock keeper waving a hand.

Lines must be tended constantly to keep the boat alongside. This means taking in slack when the water rises and letting out more line as the level falls. There should be plenty of line available for the latter. If there is sufficient time to rig a slip line this saves a crew member staying ashore to cast off when the boat is ready to leave. Always take a turn around a cleat on board when holding a mooring line in order to take the strain as there can be quite a surge in the lock due to water movement as sluice gates are operated.

If a long passage through a canal system is envisaged, a collapsible bicycle is a useful accessory to enable a crew member to go on ahead to the next lock to prepare it ready for enty.

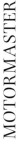
MOTORMASTER

QUESTIONS

12.1 Approaching from the south west you anticipate arriving in Dartmouth at some time after noon on 26th July. From the tide tables, high water at Dartmouth is at 1204 BST and low water at 1743 neap tides. Using extracts in Figs 6.3, 12.7 and

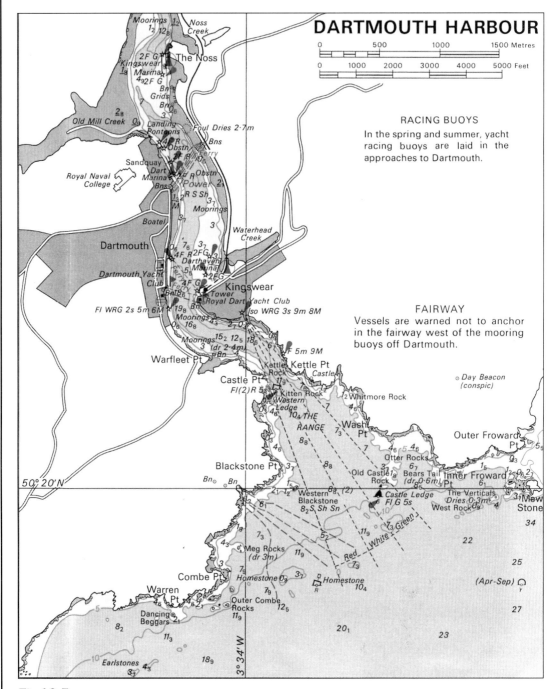

Fig 12.7

DARTMOUTH

Approach. A fine natural harbour which lies between Start Pt and Berry Head. The entrance lies between steep hills and can be difficult to distinguish but there is a conspic. daymark on the east side of the entrance. From the south, keep well clear of the Earlstones, a rocky patch with a least depth of 3.7m which lies 6 cables SW of Combe Pt. Old Combe Rk in line with Western Blackstone bearing 033°T leads east of them. There are a number of offlying rocks between Warren Pt. and Combe Pt. Western Blackstone, 2m high, lies 1 cable SE of Blackstone Pt. Homestone, with 0.9m over it is marked by a red can buoy and a rocky patch extends NW from this. From the east, there are several rocks close inshore between the Mewstone and Castle Ledge, which is marked by a lit green conical buoy which has a least depth of 1.8m LAT. It is possible with local knowledge, to pass inside the Mewstone, leaving the rocks off Froward Pt. to port.

At night, enter the harbour in the white sector of Kingswear lighthouse leaving the Castle Ledge buoy to starboard and Checkstone buoy to port. Then follow the white sector of the Bayards Cove light until the harbour opens up.

Entrance Channel. The entrance is approx. 1 cable wide between the rocks on either side and has a depth of approx. 7.9m. Once through the narrows between Kingswear Castle and Dartmouth Castle, the harbour opens out, the channel having a depth of 9m. The wind can be very fluky in the entrance.

Tidal Streams. About 1½ miles outside the entrance, streams run NE from 2 hours before to 4 hours after HW Dartmouth and SW from 2 hours before to 4 hours after LW Dartmouth. In the entrance, the stream rarely exceeds 2 knots except after heavy rainfall or strong northerly winds, when the ebb can run at up to 3½ knots.

Fig 12.8

12.8, prepare a pilotage plan for entry (a) by day, and (b) by night.

12.2 a) How would you recognise Portland Bill (i) by day, (ii) by night?
b) How does Portland Bill differ from Anvil Point (i) by day, (ii) by night?
Use Figs 12.9 and 12.10.

PORTLAND BILL 50°30.8′N, 2°27.3′W. Lt. Fl.(4) 20 sec. 29M. Shows gradually one flash to four flashes from 221° to 244°; then four flashes to 117°, gradually changing to one flash to 141°. Not vis. elsewhere. White circular Tr. with R. band near extremity of Bill. 43m. Dia. 30 sec. Window in same Lt.Ho. F.R. 13M. Vis. over Shambles Shoals from 271° to 291°. 19m. Conspicuous white beacon 18m. high at the point of the Bill.
Extreme caution necessary due to The Race (see Tidal notes).

W SHAMBLES. Lt.By. Q.(9) 15 sec. Pillar. Y.B.Y. Topmark W. Bell.
E SHAMBLES Lt.By. Q.(3) 10 sec. Pillar B.Y.B. Topmark E. w.a. Whis. ⌇.
TRIPLANE B. Lt.By. Fl. 10 sec. Sph.Y.

INSHORE WAYPOINT WEYMOUTH BAY.
50°35.0′N, 2°22.0′W.

Fig 12.9

ANVIL POINT 50°35.5′N, 1°57.5′W. Lt. Fl. 10 sec. 24M. vis. 237° to 076°. White Tr. 45m. shown H24.

PEVERIL LEDGE By. Can. R. Off Peveril Pt.

Fig 12.10

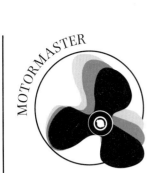

CHAPTER THIRTEEN

AUTHORITIES & NAUTICAL PUBLICATIONS

COASTGUARD

Her Majesty's Coastguard has, as its principal task, the responsibility for co-ordination of search and rescue at sea. The Coastguard generally only covers United Kingdom coastal waters out to about 30 miles offshore. Other national authorities have similar organisations responsible for the co-ordination of search and rescue within their coastal waters. Normally the Coastguard will perform a general monitoring function, but in emergencies, like the fire and ambulance services, they take absolute control and all craft must comply with their directions.

Around the UK coast Maritime Rescue Co-ordination Centres are manned by the

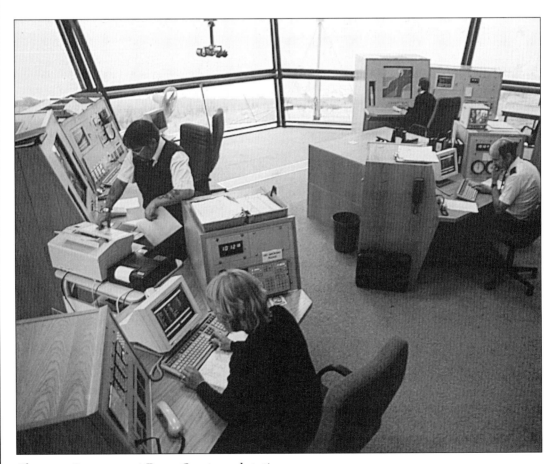

The operations room at Dover Coastguard station.

MOTORMASTER

90

Coastguard, some on a 24 hour basis. The Coastguard normally communicates with ships using VHF radio. The normal working channel is 67 after initial contact on channel 16. Occasionally channel 73 and channel 06 are used.

The Yacht and Boat Safety Scheme

Every year the Coastguard is alerted to over 1000 small craft which are either overdue or in distress. Having been alerted, one of the main difficulties is lack of detailed informa tion about these craft, such as: type, size and appearance of craft, safety equipment on board, and normal cruising area. The Yacht and Boat Safety Scheme has been set up to provide a database containing this information. This data can help to speed up a search and rescue operation.

To register for this scheme, you should complete Form CG66 obtainable from Coastguard offices, marinas, yacht clubs and harbourmasters' offices. Post the completed form together with a recent photograph of the craft, if available, to the nearest Coastguard Maritime Centre.

Whenever a passage is planned, you should leave details with someone responsible ashore who can then contact the Coastguard in the event of the boat being overdue at its destination. Do not forget to inform your shore contact that you have arrived safely.

Details of a longer passage can also be given to the Coastguard, either by making direct contact on VHF radio or by telephone ashore before leaving the harbour. If the craft is overdue, your shore contact should inform the nearest Coastguard who will then take appropriate action.

For passages outside coastal waters, contact the nearest Maritime Rescue Centre and give appropriate details. This is then available to overseas rescue organisations if needed. If you change your plan tell your contact ashore or inform the Coastguard.

Navigational warnings and weather forecasts

Navigational and strong wind warnings are broadcast by the Coastguard. You can obtain a weather forecast by telephone but it is better to listen to their regular broadcasts than contact the Coastguard direct.

Yacht Safety Information Broadcasts

At times the Coastguard may require assistance to locate other craft. This request is broadcast by VHF radio as a Yacht Safety Information Broadcast announced on channel 16 and broadcast on channel 67.

Channel Navigational Information Service

Dover Coastguard and Gris Nez Traffic on VHF channels 10 and 11 respectively operate a Channel Navigation Information Service in the Dover Straits. Broadcasts are every half hour and give details of navigational hazards in the area.

THE METEOROLOGICAL OFFICE

There are many different ways of obtaining forecasts of the weather at sea, though most are limited to a period of 24 hours

MOTORMASTER

ahead. Traditionally the shipping forecast, prepared by the London Weather Centre and broadcast by the British Broadcasting Corporation, is the basis of weather predictions for the sea areas around northwest Europe. Local weather forecasts give more up-to-the-minute information for short passages (see Chapter 21).

INTERNATIONAL MARITIME ORGANISATION (IMO)

The International Maritime Organisation (IMO) is responsible for the International Regulations for Preventing Collisions at Sea (IRPCS). The skipper of any seagoing craft must be fully aware of these regulations: they are the equivalent of the Highway Code for motorists. The Regulations cover the basic steering rules, rules covering special situations, and rules for the showing of lights and the sounding of fog signals. Further information is given in Chapter 23.

HARBOUR AUTHORITIES

Harbour and port authorities are responsible for the safety of all ship movements within their harbour and its approaches. The following points are of particular concern for skippers of small craft and the Harbour or Port authorities should be able to give you information:

- Knowledge of prohibited and restricted areas. Areas in harbours or their approaches designated for specific purposes.

- Traffic separation schemes (see page 191).

- Appreciation of ship movements within a harbour.

- Speed restrictions in operation.

- Anti–pollution regulations.

- Knowledge of the duties and obligations of the master of a vessel under Harbour bye laws, local Notices to Mariners and national legislation, and knowledge of where to obtain this information.

- Special operations within a harbour area: dredging, dumping of spoil, diving operations, loading and discharging of hazardous cargoes, etc.

- Procedures for reporting accidents.

- The use of VHF radio to monitor shipping movements within areas covered by Vessel Traffic Services (VTS) and Harbour Control.

- The ability to recognise the constraints of a large commercial vessel in a restricted narrow channel with limited under-keel clearance.

- An understanding of the interaction between ships and the need to give an adequate separation distance when overtaking, crossing or passing.

- Precautions to be observed when manoeuvring in congested waters where other vessels may be obscured by intervening obstructions.

- Precautions and actions to be taken when navigating in restricted visibility within harbour approaches.

Ideally the majority of local information is promulgated through yacht clubs and marina offices. Motorboats with an alert helmsman should have no difficulty in keeping clear of commercial shipping, but awareness is important and can best be achieved by monitoring the VHF radio port operations channel (usually either channel 12 or 14).

NAUTICAL PUBLICATIONS

The publications given below will give you information sources for pilotage and passage planning.

Nautical almanacs contain much of the information in the separate publications given below, such as lists of lights, fog signals, lists of radio signals, aids to navigation and pilotage, harbour chartlets, tide tables and tidal stream diagrams. Almanacs are re-issued annually.

Tide tables, tidal stream atlas or tidal diagrams or current charts. See Chapter 7.

List of radio signals Information includes radio regulations, marine direction finding stations, radiobeacons, Loran, Decca, radar, broadcasting frequencies and times of transmission, time signals. They are corrected by reference to Notices to Mariners.

UK Admiralty List of Radio Signals is published by the Hydrographic Office and is in several volumes. The main volumes of interest to the small boat user are: Volume 2 – Radio Navigational Aids, NP282, Volume 3 – Radio Weather Services, NP283. Coverage is worldwide.

List of lights and fog signals Information regarding lights is shown on charts but in an abbreviated form. A fuller description is given in lights lists published by various countries. Typical information is: name and location of light, latitude and longitude, characteristics, height, range, description of structure as seen by day, fog signal. The UK Admiralty List of Lights and Fog Signals is published by the Hydrographic Office and is re-issued periodically. Coverage is worldwide. All lights lists are corrected by reference to Notices to Mariners.

Sailing directions or pilots Charts give information in an abbreviated form and because they need to be understood at a glance it is not possible to incorporate very detailed information. Pilot books, on the other hand are meant to be studied beforehand and include photographs of land and sea features, anchorages, port facilities, hazards, sketches showing safe tracks, transits, harbour and river plans and tidal information.

UK Sailing Directions NP 1–72 These are published by the Hydrographic Office and coverage is worldwide. They are revised and re-issued periodically and between revisions updated by supplements.

US Coast Pilots These are published by the National Ocean Survey and consist of a number of books covering United States coastal, intercoastal and Great Lakes waters. They are published annually or bi-annually and corrected by reference to Notices to Mariners.

US Sailing Directions These cover world areas outside the United States. They are published by the Defense Mapping Agency Hydrographic/Topographic Centre. Reprints are published dependent upon the number of revisions to be incorporated.

Other countries Many maritime countries produce pilots and sailing directions published by their own hydrographic office. These local guides are often the best up-to-date source of information for the areas concerned.

The Admiralty List of Chart Symbols and Abbreviations, Chart 5011, used for British Admiralty Charts; or _Nautical Chart Symbols and Abbreviations_, Chart No 1, published in the USA by the Department of Commerce.

MOTORMASTER

NAVIGATION

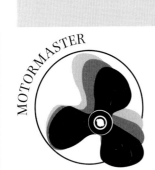

CHAPTER FOURTEEN

CHARTWORK

When driving along a motorway, you use directional signs to find your way. The length of time the journey takes depends upon the speed the car is travelling and the distance to be covered; so a car travelling at 45 miles per hour would take 2 hours 13 minutes to complete a 100 mile journey. Similarly, given an open sea, a boat motoring at 20 knots would take 5 hours to cover 100 miles. There are, of course, no signposts out of sight of land so the compass becomes the principal instrument to indicate the direction in which to steer (See Chapter 4).

You will most probably be navigating using electronic systems (see Chapter 15), but should such systems fail (which they can do if the boat experiences electrical or battery problems), you will have no choice but to resort to the traditional methods of navigation in order to reach port safely. So you need to know the basics.

COURSE TO STEER

The first thing you need to know when leaving harbour is the direction or *course to steer* towards your destination. This course is found by marking the starting position, ie the first *waypoint* on a chart, and, with plotting

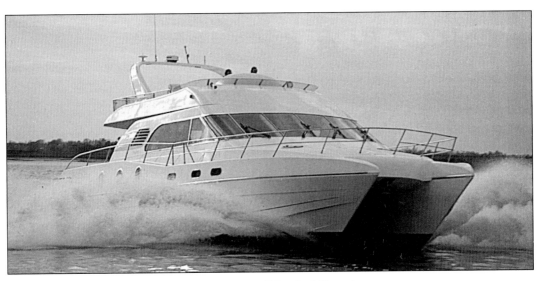

Dreamboat – this 61 foot Prout catamaran confidently follows her course.

instruments, finding the direction that the next waypoint bears from the starting position. You will also want an *estimated time of arrival* (ETA) at that waypoint. This is found by measuring the distance between the starting position and the waypoint and dividing it by the boat's anticipated speed. This *elapsed time* is added to the time of commencement of the passage to give the ETA at the waypoint. By repeating this procedure for each waypoint to the destination, the ETA at the destination can be determined.

Look at Fig 14.1. The starting point is marked as Waypoint 1 and the next waypoint as Waypoint 2 (WP1 and WP2). The direction of Waypoint 2 from Waypoint 1 is 045°T. This direction is the desired track, known as the *ground track*. The distance between the two waypoints is 15 nautical miles. This is found by reference to the scale in Fig 14.1 (see Measuring Distance in Chapter 6).

In the absence of other factors, the ground track shown in Fig 14.1 would be the *course to steer*. So a boat motoring from Waypoint 1 on a course of 045°T at 8 knots (nautical miles per hour) would arrive at Waypoint 2 in 1 hr 52 mins 30 secs:

$15 \div 8 = 1.875$ hrs

= 1 hr 52 mins 30 secs.

There are however, other factors which may affect your course. Both tidal stream and wind can cause the boat to deviate from the desired track. In a large planing motorboat with powerful engines, wind and tide are of less importance but smaller craft with displacement hulls travelling at slower speeds will need to take these factors into consideration. Also for qualification in navigational skills you will need to include allowances for tide and wind in your chartwork calculations. Some of the exercises or examples that follow are in

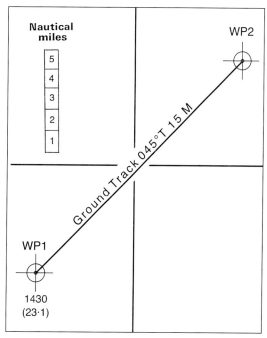

Fig 14.1 *Ground track*

areas where the tidal stream would be negligible to a high speed motorboat. Low boat speeds are used so that the principles involved can be easily understood.

Tidal stream

First we need to consider what effect the tidal stream will have on the boat.

A tidal stream directly ahead or astern of the boat will not displace the boat from the ground track, but it will affect the speed the boat is actually *making good* over the ground (ie the boat's motion relative to the land or seabed rather than the water), either decreasing it or increasing it. For example, a boat with a speed through the water of 10 knots, experiencing a 3 knot tidal stream from ahead, ie a foul tide, will only make good 7 knots over the ground, whereas the same boat travelling at 10 knots but experiencing a 3 knot tidal stream from astern, ie a fair tide, will make good 13 knots over the ground. The speed made good can be nearly doubled by using a fair tidal stream.

A tidal stream across the boat's track will both displace the boat from its ground track and affect its speed made good over the ground, unless the tidal stream is at right angles to the track, when only the boat's displacement is affected.

A boat travelling on a course of 045°T from Waypoint 1 in Figure 14.1 and experiencing a tidal stream flowing in a south-easterly direction (135°) will not reach Waypoint 2, but will pass to the south of it.

Tidal stream data is normally given on charts in the form of a table, and in a tidal stream atlas as a diagram (see Figs 7.6 and 7.17 in Chapter 7).

Wind

Wind has a similar effect upon the boat as the tidal stream. If it is ahead or astern it will not cause sideways displacement, but may affect the boat's speed.

When the wind is across the boat's track, it acts on the superstructure, causing a sideways deflection known as leeway angle or, more simply, as *leeway*. The direction of the deflection is away from the direction from which the wind is blowing, so a boat travelling on a course of 045°T as in Fig 14.1, and experiencing a northwesterly wind causing 5° of leeway, would not reach Waypoint 2, but would be deflected to the south. As the speed of the boat increases, the effective leeway is reduced.

Strong winds can cause heavy disturbed seas which are uncomfortable and may be dangerous. Chapter 20 on Weather Systems explains the effects in more detail.

Allowing for tidal stream and wind

As we have seen, unless allowances are made for the effects of tidal stream and wind the boat will not remain on the desired ground track to reach the destination. To find the course to steer, you have to plot a *vector diagram* on the chart. The procedure is as follows:

1 Plot Waypoint 1 and 2, and draw a line from one to the other. This is the ground track on which the boat must stay in order to reach Waypoint 2. Write the time of departure (1430) and the log reading (how far you have already travelled in nautical miles) in brackets (23.1) beside Waypoint 1 (Fig 14.1).

2 Measure the distance between the two waypoints (15 nautical miles).

3 The boat's speed is 8 knots. Estimate approximately how long it will take to reach Waypoint 2, ignoring for the moment the tidal stream. This will be nearly 2 hours. For plotting purposes we will assume a passage time of 2 hours.

4 Check the tidal streams, we will assume that the tidal stream for the first hour is 110°T 1.5 kn, and for the second hour 100°T 1.2 kn. The tidal stream will displace the boat to the south but as it is slightly astern of the boat, the elapsed time of the passage will be shorter than the initial assessment.

5 Plot from Waypoint 1 the tidal stream vector for the first hour (110°T 1.5 kn). At the end of this vector, plot the tidal stream vector for the second hour (100°T 1.2 kn). *Note*: for a tidal stream of 240° 1.8kn, the distance travelled over a period of 30 mins (say) would be 0.9 nautical miles ie plot 240° 0.9M. Fig 14.2 shows this.

6 The boat's speed is 8 knots through the water. The vector diagram is being plotted for a period of 2 hours, so we have plotted 2 hours of tidal stream. The boat

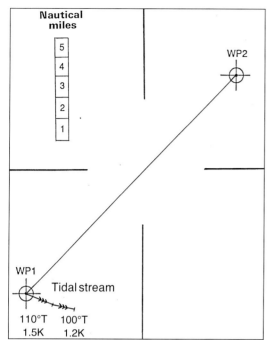

Fig 14.2 *Allowing for two hours of tidal stream*

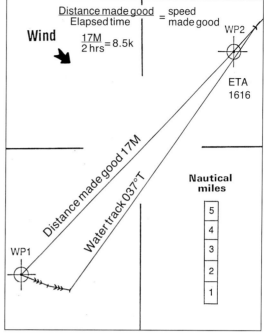

Fig 14.3 *Water track*

will travel 8 miles through the water in one hour, so for a period of 2 hours, we will need to plot a distance of 16 miles. This is measured from the latitude scale down the side of the chart using dividers.

7 Keeping the dividers 16 miles apart, place one point of the dividers at the end of the second hour of the tidal stream vector and move the other point of the dividers to intersect the ground track, extended if necessary. Mark this position, which should be fairly close to Waypoint 2. Draw a line from the end of the tidal stream vector to this position, Fig 14.3.

8 This line is the track of the boat through the water, known as the *water track*. Its direction is measured as 037°T. The water track allows for tidal stream but not for leeway caused by the wind.

9 The boat is experiencing a northwesterly wind causing 5° of leeway. To allow for

this, the measured water track is corrected by applying an adjustment of 5° towards the direction of the wind. This is not plotted but is done arithmetically by subtracting the 5° from 037°T. The resultant figure is the course to steer, which is 032°T. The course to steer allows for tidal stream and wind.

10 The distance the boat has actually travelled in two hours is that distance measured from Waypoint 1 to the marked position on the ground track. This is called the distance made good over the ground, or *distance made good*. The distance made good is 17 nautical miles.

11 The speed made good over the ground, or *speed made good*, is found by dividing the distance made good by the time of two hours. The speed made good is 8.5 kn.

12 Our initial assessment of the passage time between the waypoints was two hours. If the exact elapsed time is

MOTORMASTER

required, this can be determined by dividing the distance to go from Waypoint 1 to Waypoint 2 (15 miles) by the speed made good (8.5 knots). This will give 1 hr 46 mins, making the ETA at Waypoint 2 to be 1616.

FIXING POSITION

Your position found by reference to land-marks and seamarks, such as a lighthouse or a radiobeacon, or measured by an electronic navigation system (Decca or GPS), is called a *fix*. A fix is not dependent upon the boat's course, distance run, lee-way or tidal stream, and is normally quite precise.

Three position line fix

Fig 14.4 shows a fix obtained by using three compass bearings of landmarks. These bearings, when plotted on a chart, are known as *position lines*. The point of intersection of these position lines is the boat's fixed position at the time of taking the bearings. The symbol used for a fix is ⊙. The time that the fix was taken and the log reading are written on the chart adja-cent to the fix.

Usually the position lines do not inter-sect exactly but form a small triangle known as a *cocked hat*. If the cocked hat is large it shows that the compass readings were not very accurate, so the bearings should be checked and possibly retaken.

Errors causing a cocked hat:

- Inaccuracy when taking the bearings.

- Bad plotting.

- Variation incorrectly applied.

- One or more objects incorrectly identified.

- The distance the boat has travelled between bearings.

Two position line fix

A fix obtained from the use of two bearings is not as reliable as one using three posi-tion lines as there is no cocked hat to show up any error. However, if there is a good angle (around 90°) between the position lines, quite good results can be obtained. Sometimes, of course, there may be only two landmarks available from which to take bearings.

Selection of marks for position fixing

The following points should be considered when choosing marks to provide position lines:

- When two position lines are used, the angle between them should be approxi-mately 90°. When three position lines are used the angle between them should be about 60°.

- Nearer marks are preferred. The greater the distance away, the greater the possi-bility of error.

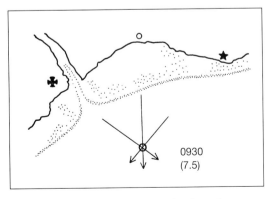

Fig 14.4 *A plotted position fix from bearings on three objects. The intersection is rarely as accurate as this.*

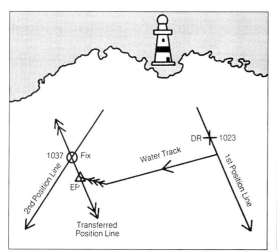

Fig 14.5 *The transferred position line, which should be plotted with double arrowheads at each end.*

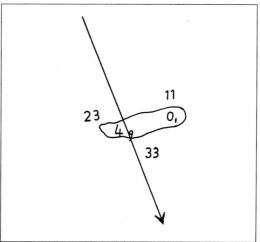

Fig 14.6 *A single position line crossing a sounding on an isolated shoal.*

- Bearings ahead or astern should be taken first as they only change slowly. Bearings abeam can alter rapidly so they are taken last.

- Left-hand and right-hand edges of cliffs can be used for bearings provided they are steep.

- At night, lights must be positively identified from their characteristics.

SOUNDINGS

On a chart the depth of water below chart datum is given in figures (usually in metres) called soundings. We can use this information to help us to fix our position. We measure the depth of water under the boat by using an echo sounder. (The depth measured is actually between the seabed and the sensor or transducer mounted on the boat's hull). The depth of water, when corrected for the height of tide, will correspond with the soundings shown on the chart. A sounding of a prominent feature on the seabed can be used together with a position line from another source to indicate the boat's position, Fig 14.6.

Depth contours

We have already seen (Chapter 5 Fig 5.8) that a line on a chart joining points of equal depth is called a *contour line*. If this contour line is fairly straight it can be used as an underwater position line or as an indication of the edge of the channel. By following a depth contour (altering course to remain in a constant water depth) it is frequently possible to skirt round an underwater hazard in conditions of poor visibility.

DEAD RECKONING POSITION

Dead Reckoning position (DR) is an approximate position deduced from the course steered and distance run and taking no account of wind and tidal stream. It is plotted on the chart using the symbol +. It forms the basis for calculating the more accurate Estimated Position.

ESTIMATED POSITION

If you cannot work out your position by taking fixes, then the boat's position can be estimated by constructing a vector diagram as follows:

1 A boat has been travelling at a speed of 10 knots on a course of 060°T for a period of 1 hr 30 mins (Fig 14.7). The distance run is 15M.

2 The boat may have been displaced laterally from the course steered by the effect of the wind. This displacement will have been away from the direction of the wind. If the wind direction was from the southeast and the leeway was estimated at 5°, the boat will have been pushed towards the northwest at an angle of 5°. Leeway is applied arithmetically to give the water track which is 055°T. This water track is plotted from Waypoint 1

for the distance run of 15M. The departure time (0900) and the distance travelled (log reading 45.4) is marked beside Waypoint 1, Fig 14.8.

3 We then need to take account of the tide. The tidal stream experienced during the passage time of 1 hr 30 mins is plotted at the end of the water track. Look up the tidal streams. Assume that the tidal stream for the first hour was in the direction of 295°T at a speed of 2.5 knots, so we use our plotter to mark this direction for 2.5M ie the distance the tide will have taken us in an hour (2.5M plotted) and for the second hour, 330°T 2.2 knots (only 30 minutes needed so 1.1M plotted), Fig 14.9.

4 The position at the end of the tidal streams is marked with the symbol △ and the time and log reading placed next to it. This is an *estimated position* (EP). It is not as accurate as a fix of position,

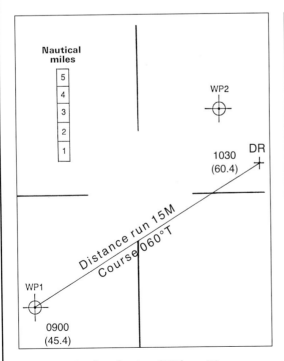

Fig 14.7 *Dead reckoning (DR) position*

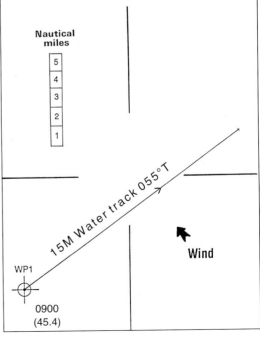

Fig 14.8 *Water track allows for leeway*

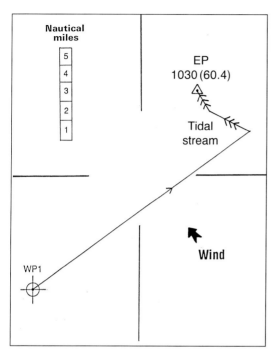

Fig 14.9 *Estimated position*

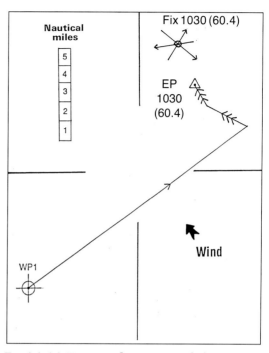

Fig 14.10 *Estimated position with fix.*

because it relies upon wind and tidal stream estimations which are often incorrect. (Fig 14.10, by comparison, shows the fix of the boat's position which is some distance away from the estimated position.)

5 The boat's track over the ground (*ground track*) is from Waypoint 1 to the estimated position. It is not necessary to plot the ground track.

Transferred position line

When there is only one landmark or seamark available for position fixing, the following method can be used to fix the position of the boat, Fig 14.5. (See Estimated Position above.)

1 Take a bearing of the mark and plot the resultant position line.

2 After a period of time sufficient to give a good angle between the position lines, obtain a second bearing of the mark.

3 For the period of time between bearings, plot the water track. This can be plotted from *any* point on the first position line.

4 At the end of the water track, plot the tidal stream for the same time period as the water track and thus obtain the estimated position.

5 Plot the second position line.

6 Transfer the first position line so that it passes through the estimated position and intersects the second position line.

The point of intersection of the transferred position line and the second position line is the position fix. Ideally the two position lines should cut at 90°. The accuracy of a transferred position line depends upon:

- Correct estimation of water track.
- Correct assessment of tidal stream.
- Accurate bearings.
- Accurate distance run.

COMPARISON OF METHODS TO DETERMINE POSITION

Dead Reckoning The position obtained from the course steered and distance run. Not accurate.

Estimated Position The best estimate of the boat's position taking into account the course steered, distance run and the effects of tidal stream and wind. Better than a dead reckoning position but not as good as a fix.

Transferred Position Line Useful when only one mark is visible at any one time. Only as accurate as the assessment of the water track, distance run and tidal stream.

Soundings Measuring the depth of water. The approximate position of the boat must be known. Unless there is prominent unmistakable feature on the seabed a sounding only gives a rough indication of position. Accuracy is improved if soundings are used with a position line from another source.

Distance off by Dipping Light (See page 71.) A useful method when making a landfall by night. Not accurate.

Single Position Line One position line only indicates that the boat's position lies somewhere along it.

Two or more visual bearings Two bearings are very accurate provided that there is a good angle of cut between the position lines. The best fix is by three visual bearings whose position lines intersect at about 60° to each other.

Positions from electronic navigation systems Potentially very accurate.

Close inshore, there may not be time to fix the boat's position. A leading line (transit) allows you to appreciate rapidly any tendency for the boat to be set off track; clearing bearings also useful because they help ensure that navigational hazards are avoided (see Chapter 11). An echo sounder should always be used to verify position.

With reliable electronic fixing systems, a position can be obtained at any time and so it is not necessary (nor is it practical, on a fast moving boat) to take visual bearings with a hand-bearing compass or to plot estimated positions. However, should there be a system failure, as mentioned above, it may be necessary to reduce speed and use these basic methods.

QUESTIONS

Use a variation of 5°W and the Deviation Table shown in Fig 4.4, Chapter 4. All times British Summer Time (BST). Use the section of Stanfords chart No 12 shown in Fig 14.11 and the associated tidal stream data in Fig 14.12.

14.1 The boat's position at 1430 is 50° 07′N 3° 49′W. Course 052°C. Leeway 5° due to northwest wind. Boat's speed is 8kn. High water Plymouth is at 1600, springs.
a) What is the boat's estimated position at 1530?

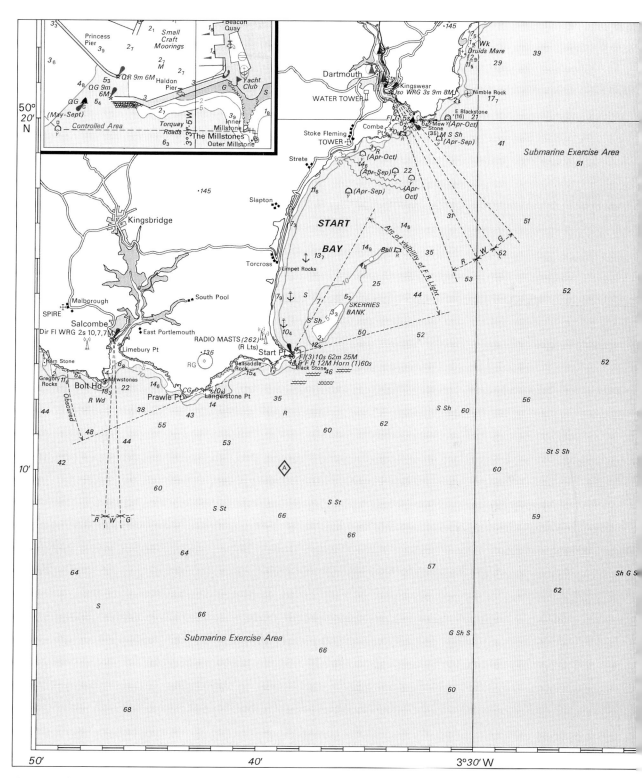

Figure 14.11

Tidal Steams referred to HW at PLYMOUTH (Devonport)

Hours		A 50°10'·0N 3 38·8W Dir	Rate (kn) Sp	Np	B 50°18'·0N 3.20·0W Dir	Rate (kn) Sp	Np	C 50°29'·3N 2 57·5W Dir	Rate (kn) Sp	Np	D 50°29'·6N 2 26.6W Dir	Rate (kn) Sp	Np	E 50°26'·3N 2 26.4W Dir	Rate (kn) Sp	Np	F 50°28'·3N 1 59.7W Dir	Rate (kn) Sp	Np	G 50°35'·5N 1 38.5W Dir	Rate (kn) Sp	Np	Hours	
Before HW	6	245	1·3	0·7	227	1·0	0·5	252	0·7	0·4	249	7·0	3·5	263	1·5	0·7	261	1·2	0·6	264	1·3	0·7	6	Before HW
	5	243	2·0	1·0	232	1·4	0·7	265	1·3	0·6	240	7·0	3·5	270	2·8	1·4	258	2·5	1·2	266	2·0	1·1	5	
	4	241	2·1	1·0	234	1·5	0·7	271	1·3	0·6	236	6·4	3·2	267	3·6	1·8	252	3·4	1·7	265	2·2	1·3	4	
	3	244	1·3	0·7	241	0·8	0·4	281	0·9	0·5	228	4·8	2·4	261	3·0	1·5	252	3·0	1·5	265	1·8	1·0	3	
	2	206	0·3	0·2	307	0·3	0·1	306	0·4	0·2	219	2·0	1·0	258	1·5	0·7	250	1·8	0·9	267	1·0	0·6	2	
	1	066	1·0	0·5	034	0·7	0·3	029	0·4	0·2	112	0·9	0·5	158	0·2	0·1	296	0·5	0·3	350	0·2	0·1	1	
HW		062	1·6	0·8	048	1·1	0·6	059	0·7	0·3	111	4·5	2·2	105	1·6	0·8	057	1·0	0·5	076	0·9	0·5	HW	
After HW	1	059	2·0	1·0	055	1·4	0·7	067	0·9	0·5	102	5·6	2·8	101	2·8	1·4	074	2·1	1·0	084	1·5	0·8	1	After HW
	2	053	1·8	0·9	061	1·4	0·7	074	1·1	0·5	109	4·6	2·3	101	3·6	1·8	078	2·9	1·4	087	2·0	1·1	2	
	3	060	1·0	0·5	060	0·8	0·4	081	1·1	0·5	119	3·8	1·9	108	3·7	1·8	074	2·8	1·4	089	2·0	1·1	3	
	4	100	0·3	0·2	074	0·3	0·2	093	0·7	0·4	138	2·7	1·3	117	2·2	1·1	081	2·0	1·0	091	1·4	0·8	4	
	5	226	0·5	0·3	201	0·2	0·1	136	0·3	0·2	209	2·2	1·1	121	0·7	0·3	074	0·7	0·3	098	0·6	0·3	5	
	6	248	1·1	0·5	222	0·8	0·4	229	0·4	0·2	247	5·2	2·6	261	1·0	0·5	283	0·6	0·3	257	0·7	0·4	6	

Fig 14.12

b) If the same course is maintained, will the boat clear the overfalls to the south-east of Start Point?

14.2   At 1030 the boat's position is 127°T Start Point lighthouse 217°M. Course 222°C. Leeway 5° due to southeast wind. Boat speed 10kn. High water Plymouth 1600, neaps. What is the boat's estimated position at 1130?

14.3   a)   At 0430 a boat takes a bearing of Start Point light of 245°M just as the Iso WRG 3s sectored light at Kingswear (Dartmouth) changes from white to red. What is the boat's position? Is this a good fix?
b) High water Plymouth is at 0400 spring tides. The course set is 197°C. Boat speed 9kn. Leeway nil. What is the boat's estimated position at 0600?

14.4   At 1615 a boat, in DR position 50° 15'N 3° 31'W, sights Start Point lighthouse on a bearing of 265°M. She continues on her course of 217°C at a speed of 12 knots. At 1645 Start Point lighthouse bears 351°M. High water Plymouth 1530, springs. Leeway nil. What is the boat's position at 1645?

14.5   At 1720 a motor boat heading for Salcombe gets a Decca fix of 50° 02.5'N 3°31'W. The boat speed is 11 knots. High water Plymouth 1550, springs. Leeway nil. What is the compass course to steer for a position 216°T Prawle Point 1.0M? What is the ETA at this position?

14.6   At 0730 a motor boat is in a position 1M south of Bolt Head making a speed of 18 knots. High water Plymouth 1245, springs. No leeway. What is the compass course to steer and the ETA at the waypoint position 50° 03'N 3° 40'W?

14.7   A boat leaves Dartmouth just after 0400 at a speed of 8 knots. At 0500 the Decca gives a warning 'Position suspect'. At that time the Decca reads 50° 18.47'N 3° 32.56'W. At that moment the navigator observes the Iso WRG 3s light at Kingswear change from white to red and the F R light on Start Point go out. The course is 155°C. Is the Decca position correct? If not, what is the correct position?

MOTORMASTER

CHAPTER FIFTEEN

ELECTRONIC NAVIGATION SYSTEMS

WHAT IS ELECTRONIC NAVIGATION?

An electronic position–finding system, such as Decca, Loran or GPS, provided it is working satisfactorily, can give a constant read-out of the boat's present position, usually to an accuracy of 100 m. In visual navigation, the present position is based on a fix from two or three position lines obtained from bearings of landmarks taken with the hand-bearing compass. An electronic system does not require a landmark to be visible. Systems based on radio waves transmitted from shore stations, known as hyperbolic systems, provide accurate present positions in all weather conditions, but their range is limited. Systems based on radio signals transmitted from satellites will give the equivalent accuracy but with global coverage.

Waypoints for position-finding

In all position-finding systems the first objective is to establish the boat's position, and additional selected positions, ie *waypoints*, can be entered. For example, by entering the latitude and longitude of a series of buoys as waypoints, so that as each one is passed, the next can be selected, you can readily appreciate exactly where you are. If the buoys are identified by highlighting on the chart, then no separate plotting is necessary which can save much trouble at high speeds or in rough seas. This method is only realistic if the passage planning (see Chapter 25) has been completed properly and the appropriate waypoints entered in the electronic receiver.

Course and speed made good can also be displayed, as well as cross track error (ie the distance you are off course and which way to move the helm to get back on course) and estimated time of arrival (ETA) at destination. Man overboard position markers (MOB) are sometimes included. Some systems will work out tidal stream or current if the boat's course and speed are entered.

Using charts

Electronic means of navigation need to be used in conjunction with charts. Paper charts, whilst they are ideal for passage planning, are difficult to use in a high speed craft. They are now being complemented by electronic charts, the scale of which can be instantly adjusted to your requirements and, when linked to an electronic position finding system, can be used to display the boat's position relative to adjacent coastlines and hazards to navigation.

It is not necessary to know how the various electronic systems work as long as the capabilities and limitations are clearly understood. You should be able to identify readily any system failure so that a back-up manual system can be quickly adopted. Traditionally, positions, courses and speeds are entered regularly in the *deck log*. In high speed craft a paper printout of position, course and speed made good at regular intervals (20 minutes) will serve as a navigational deck log rendering reversion to manual navigation a simple task.

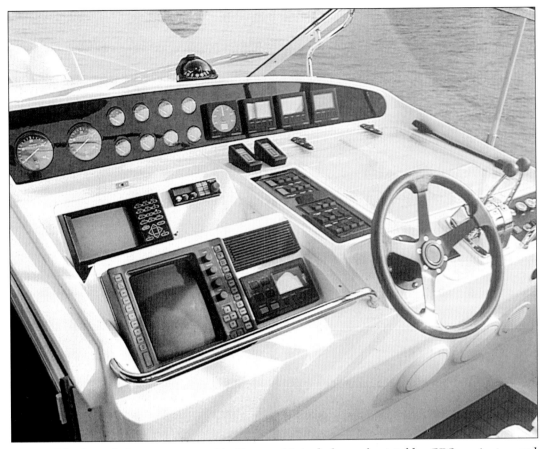

The well laid out helm position on this Broom 41 includes a chart table, GPS navigator and electronic chart display.

HYPERBOLIC NAVIGATION SYSTEMS

Hyperbolic navigation systems have now largely been superseded by GPS (Global Positioning System) which uses orbiting satellites for positioning. However, you may have inherited a Decca set with your boat or have been offered a very good second-hand deal – you can rest assured that hyperbolic systems are still very effective nav aids. So, for the technically-minded, here is a brief explanation of how they work.

Radio waves are emitted from a land based transmitter like ripples from a pond. If a vessel is midway between two such trans-

mitters with synchronised transmissions on the same radio frequency, then the peaks and troughs of the radio waves (or pulses) will be received at the same time: they are said to be *in-phase*. If the vessel is slightly nearer one transmitter than the other, then the waves or pulses from the nearer transmitter will be received first and the waves or pulses are *out-of-phase*. It is possible to measure very accurately the degree to which they are out-of-phase: this is known as phase difference for radio waves and time difference for pulses. If a series of points are plotted for positions where the difference in the distances of the two transmitters is constant (ie the phase or time difference is

MOTORMASTER

constant), then these points will form a curve known as a hyperbola.

Knowing the phase or time difference between two transmissions enables a *line of position* (LOP) to be determined. With a separate pair of transmitters a second line of position can be determined, their point of intersection being the boat's present position (Fig 15.1).

The radio receiver, though it can measure accurately the phase difference, cannot determine the whole number of cycles in the phase difference between two wave transmissions. The position lines produced by continuous wave hyperbolic systems are ambiguous because of this inability to distinguish between one *lane* and another. Within a given lane, however, there is no ambiguity and repeated visits to a given position will give the same fractional reading each time. It is as though you can tell which pew you are sitting in, but not which church. The solution to this problem is to intersperse the transmissions with signals at a lower frequency in order to establish *lane identification*.

Hyperbolic systems consist of a number of *chains*. At the centre of each chain is a master transmitter, with two or three slave (or secondary) transmitters some distance away (approximately 100 nautical miles for Decca, 300 nautical miles for Loran and 4000 nautical miles for Omega). The pattern of hyperbolic curves obtained from the pairs consisting of the master transmitter and one slave are known as a *lattice*. In the regions between transmitters, the lattice is compact and the positional accuracy is high (in the region of 50 metres). The accuracy reduces as the lattice pattern opens up, Fig 15.1. If the baseline from the master transmitter to any slave transmitter is extended beyond that slave, then the lattice becomes very open and the positional accuracy very poor.

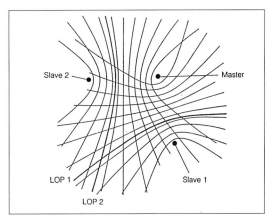

Fig 15.1 *Lines of position obtained from two pairs of transmitting stations.*

The radio receivers use the groundwave transmission from the master and slave stations which extends about 500 nautical miles. The portion of the transmission going upwards is known as the skywave. The skywave can bounce off the ionosphere returning to the earth's surface some 400 nautical miles away in daytime and 250 miles away at night when the ionosphere descends. For the Decca system the interference between the groundwave and the skywave becomes the limit to its coverage. The Loran system can switch from groundwave to skywave operation thus extending its range and reducing the problem of interference.

Decca Navigator

The Decca Navigator coverage in North West Europe is from the north of Norway to the south of Spain including the Baltic Sea. Other Decca chains are established in the Persian Gulf, Japan, South Africa, North East Canada, Nigeria, North West Australia, North West India and Bangladesh. The coverage is 400 nautical miles from the master transmitter by day and 250 nautical miles by night. Within 50 nautical miles of the transmitters an accuracy of 50 metres can be expected, but it can deteriorate considerably at night. Unreliable position indications can occur in areas between chains and on baseline extensions.

Loran C

Loran C coverage is the North and North West Atlantic, the North Pacific and the western Mediterranean. An accuracy of 200 metres can be expected out to a range of 500 nautical miles, but this improves to 70 metres at closer distances. Use of the skywave reflections from the ionosphere enables Loran C to be effective at ranges out to 1000 nautical miles and reduces its proneness to deterioration of performance at night.

Omega

Omega operates at a very low frequency (10.2 kHz) with a very long baseline (4000 to 6000 miles) between transmitters. This means it is essentially a worldwide system. Accuracy varies from 1 mile in the North Atlantic to 6 miles in the more remote parts of other oceans. Errors are at their maximum during night hours.

SATELLITE NAVIGATION

For worldwide position fixing, the use of radio broadcasts from orbiting navigation satellites is by far the most effective. The principal satellite system is the Global Positioning System (GPS) funded initially by the US Navy. The accuracy is potentially extremely high (20 m) but for security reasons standard commercially available sets have an accuracy of about 100 m (see Differential GPS on page 110). GPS operates for 24 hours a day, worldwide in any weather conditions.

Global Positioning System (GPS)

A network of 24 satellites orbit the earth at a height of 11,000M with their orbital plane at 55° to the Equator. The satellites transmit continuously to earth on two frequencies in the D band (1 to 2 GHz) and supply receivers with their position, velocity and time. Time is obtained from four atomic clocks which are so accurate that they will gain or lose only one second in 50,000 years. The satellites have an elaborate control system. There are five ground control monitor stations located around the Earth to receive technical telemetered data from the satellites. The master control station sifts all the information it receives and transmits to the satellites their own true positions in space and the satellites in turn transmit their positions to the ground users' receivers.

Typically a small craft will have a two-channel receiver. To use the receiver, switch it on and enter DR position, course and speed, and ship's time. The receiver then searches for available satellites, selects the most suitable, and starts tracking them. From each such satellite it receives the satel-

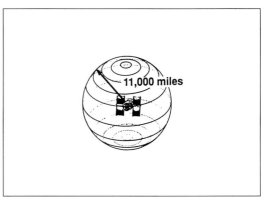

Fig 15.2

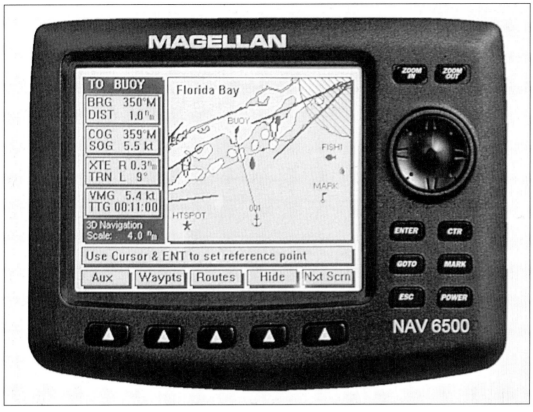

If your budget runs to it, a GPS receiver combined with a chart plotter will make navigation easier. By courtesy of Magellan Systems Corporation.

lite's position, its number and accurate time. The receiver then calculates the satellite's range by measuring the time of receipt of the signal and multiplying the time taken for the signal to come from the satellite by the speed of radio waves in air.

The receiver has thus located itself on a position sphere of known radius whose

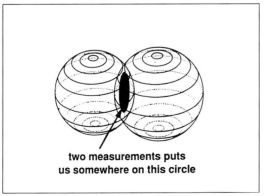

two measurements puts us somewhere on this circle

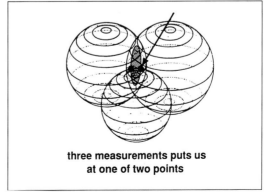

three measurements puts us at one of two points

Fig 15.3

Fig 15.4

centre is the first transmitting satellite, Fig 15.2. The receiver then measures the range of the second satellite to define a second position sphere, Fig 15.3. When a third position sphere is added, then the receiver's position is narrowed down to two points in space, Fig 15.4. As one of these two points is either many thousands of miles away from the surface of the earth or moving at a very high velocity, the computer can easily resolve which point is correct; or it could take a range measurement from a fourth satellite. The receiver can work out the point at which the position spheres intersect and display that point as latitude and longitude. For non-maritime operations, height above sea level is an additional output.

The calculation assumes that the receiver's clock is perfectly synchronised with those in the satellites. If there is an error of as little as one millisecond, there will be a range error of 163 miles resulting in a huge three-dimensional version of a 'cocked hat', Figs 15.5 and 15.6. The computer will adjust the clock time, which affects all measured ranges by the same amount, until the position spheres meet in a perfect pin-point fix.

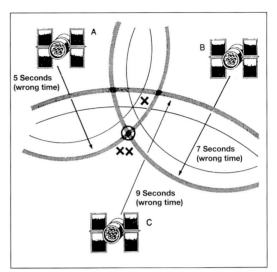

Fig 15.6 *A fixed time error is added to each position sphere giving a cocked hat and an erroneous position (XX).*

More sophisticated receivers have four or five channels which enable satellites to be tracked simultaneously giving improved accuracy and response and eliminating the need to enter a DR position on start-up.

Differential GPS

GPS was originally developed by the US government for military use. To prevent it being used against them by hostile forces, a 100 metre error was deliberately introduced when the system became commercially available. A decoder could be bought and a subscription paid to increase the accuracy. However, land-based stations have been built in Europe to correct the error – a system known as Differential GPS. This system is, however, not necessary for navigation of small craft.

RADIOBEACONS

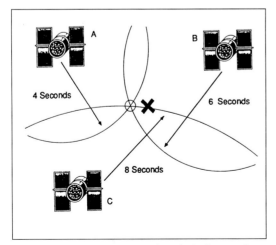

Fig 15.5 *A pin–point fix (X) from three satellites.*

A marine radiobeacon is marked on the chart with a magenta symbol. ⊙ᴿᶜ

An aeronautical radiobeacon is marked on the chart with the symbol: ⊙ *Aero RC*

A radio direction finder or RDF is used to identify and obtain a bearing of a radiobeacon provided it is within range. This bearing can then be used as a position line for a fix.

Yachtsman's almanacs contain a list of radiobeacons showing their position, frequency, identity signal, transmission time and range. Marine radiobeacons normally transmit within a period of a minute the identity signal (repeated several times), a continuous tone, and then the identity signal again. With the radio direction finder tuned to the correct frequency, the user first identifies the radiobeacon then rotates the antenna in the horizontal plane during the period of the continuous tone until the signal level drops to a minimum (known as a 'null'). The bearing is read from the magnetic compass on the antenna at the instant of the null. Whilst bearings of radiobeacons are being taken, the helmsman must try to steer a steady course.

There is a null when the antenna is directly towards the radiobeacon and when it is pointing directly away. It is usually quite evident which is the correct bearing if the radiobeacon is on the coastline. For a radiobeacon on an island or lightship, set a temporary course at right angles to the bearing of the radiobeacon: if the bearing increases the radiobeacon is on the starboard side; if it decreases the radiobeacon is to port.

An aeronautical radiobeacon transmits the continuous tone with the identity signals superimposed and without any breaks.

The radio beam is refracted (bent) when it passes either from land to sea or at a narrow angle to the coast so any bearings obtained under these conditions may be unreliable. Radio distortion frequently occurs at the time of dusk and dawn. It is not easy without practice to obtain a good bearing of a radiobeacon.

Marine radiobeacons are often used to mark the entrance to a harbour. Some radiobeacons transmit coded information about the current weather, sea and tide conditions. Others are used to carry Differential GPS data.

INTEGRATED NAVIGATION SYSTEMS

High speed cruising

High speed navigation has its own problems that differ significantly from the more sedate speeds below 15 knots. In small craft the motion of the boat, coupled with the contracted time and space available, makes the normal functions associated with navigation difficult if not impossible. At 30 knots a buoy sighted 1 mile ahead will be reached in 2 minutes.

The availability of a series of navigation sensors, each with their own display does not, however, give the navigator the solution he requires, so a logical development is to integrate the position sensor inputs with radar and electronic charts to provide a real time picture of the navigation situation. The problem then becomes a matter of trusting the displayed information and its verification.

Visual verification

At high speeds the principal danger to small craft is hitting an object floating in the water. It is important, therefore, that inboard distractions to the helmsman and navigator are reduced to a minimum. The navigator should be continually verifying the pre-planned position.

Passing close to a buoy is an obvious check on the position without the aid of

MOTORMASTER

any instruments. Other clues that can be used include judging distances and bearings, passing an identifiable landmark, evidence of breakers on a shoal, and sighting shipping lanes and ferry routes; none of them is particularly precise, but enough to cause concern if they are not seen in the right position or at the right time.

Electronic verification

The simplest electronic warning device is the echo-sounder. It can be set to sound an alarm when a set depth is reached. At other times the depth can be compared with the expected charted depth. If an electronic chart display is being used, an alarm can be set to sound when there is a significant discrepancy between actual and charted depths.

If the boat has been steering a steady course at a steady speed, then the track shown on an electronic chart display will follow a predictable line. Any deviation from this line will act as a warning; check the autopilot or the helmsman. If the track disappears off screen or stops tracking, it may be that the position fixing system has failed. If the displayed track starts to weave about it probably indicates that the received signal strength is weak or the juxtaposition of transmitting stations is giving an ambiguous result.

An ideal combination is to have the electronic chart display and the radar display side by side on the same range scale and with the radar operating in the north-up mode. This direct comparison between two independent displays can be very reassuring, particularly at night or in fog. In these conditions, steering by autopilot is preferred because of the much more stable picture the radar presents. (It is feasible but not practical to superimpose the radar display on the electronic chart display.)

A more sophisticated approach is to have duplicate electronics systems. Some position-fixing receivers have sensors for both hyperbolic and satellite networks. If by comparison the two output positions are different, then a decision has to be made which one to believe. Aircraft systems operate in triplicate with the odd one out being rejected. The dead reckoning (DR) position, obtained by input of course and speed, could be used as a third output in small craft.

Electronic chart display and information systems (ECDIS)

Once a high speed passage has begun, the use of paper charts becomes impractical. Electronic charts are available for all popular cruising areas giving fingertip access to navigational data. As electronic chart displays become more sophisticated, the result is a more user-friendly integrated navigation system. The electronic chart display enables a route to be planned on the display screen and for the boat's track to be displayed using the input position data. The display will also show other navigational information on current position, waypoints, boat speed and heading, depth, course made good, speed made good, estimated time of arrival and cross track error. It can also compute true wind direction and speed. Linked to the autopilot, a track set up on the display can be followed by the boat. With a printer connected, a printed log can be maintained every 20 minutes showing time, latitude and longitude, course made good and distance made good.

Chart plotters

For motor cruisers with displacement or semi-displacement hulls or planing cruisers under stable conditions, a chart plotter such as the Yeoman Navigator may be sufficient. By securing a paper chart to an electronic backing pad, the 'puck' control can be

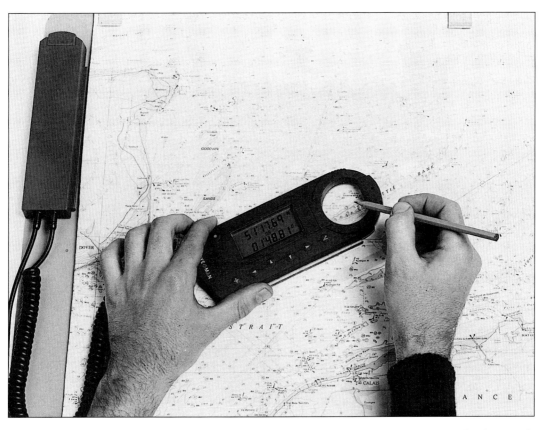

The Yeoman navigator chart plotter uses a paper chart secured to an electronic backing pad. Shown here is the 'puck' control which registers waypoints without dividers or course plotters.

moved to selected waypoints without the need for dividers and course plotting instruments, (see photo above). By connecting the puck to the output of an electronic position fixing system, the current position can be marked on the chart very simply.

RADAR

The main purpose of radar, as fitted in larger vessels, is collision avoidance. The International Regulations for Preventing Collisions at Sea states (Rule 7(b)) 'Proper use shall be made of radar equipment if fitted and operational, including long-range scanning to obtain early warning of risk of collision and radar plotting or equivalent systematic observation of detected objects.' and (Rule 7(c)) 'Assumptions shall not be made on the basis of scanty information, especially scanty radar information.' This says effectively that any vessel fitted with operational radar must use it properly if visibility deteriorates; at least one member of the crew must therefore know how to operate and plot with radar.

An increasing number of small craft have radar installed as an aid to navigation and collison avoidance as the occasion demands. There are, however, a number of problems with the installation of radar in a small craft: the screen is small (and generally lacks the definition of the showroom model); the scanner installation is

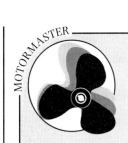

MOTORMASTER

HOW TO SET UP AN ELECTRONIC POSITION INDICATING SYSTEM

This is done in two phases:

The planning stage – entering waypoints

1 From the chart, make a list of the latitude and longitude of all the waypoints to be used in your cruise.

2 Switch on Decca or Global Positioning System (GPS) and select Waypoint Entry Mode. Enter as many waypoints as the system will allow in the order that you will reach them. Some systems have a Sail Plan Entry which enables the order of use of the waypoints to be changed.

3 Errors in waypoint entry is quite common. Use the Waypoint to Waypoint facility on the system to check that the range and bearing is compatible with that on the chart.

4 If several charts are being used, it is a good idea to mark a waypoint at the point where the next chart should be selected.

Before departure

1 Switch on Decca or GPS.

2 Check that initialisation programme is complete and that the system has achieved a lock on the boat's position.

This should be automatic but occasionally, manual entries are necessary.

3 Adjust brightness, co–ordinates of initial position, audio and visual alarms.

4 Check signal strength and waypoint sequence.

5 Check operation of Man Overboard marker.

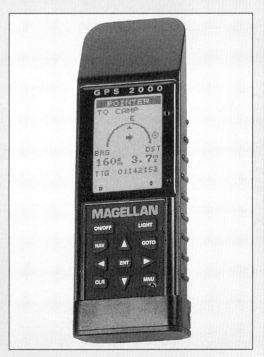

A hand-held GPS receiver. By courtesy of Magellan Systems Corporation.

cramped and low down; and the battery load can be significant. In practice radar operation and plotting is not straightforward so it is advisable to attend a one day course.

Collision avoidance

The radar echo of another vessel on a collision course remains on a steady bearing on the radar screen. The use of a chinagraph pencil to mark the echo will show how close the approaching vessel is likely to pass. By marking the echo every 6 minutes (one tenth of an hour) an estimate of the rate of approach can be determined (one mile in 6 minutes equals 10 knots). A large vessel may be detected up to 8 miles distant, but a small craft may be within 3 miles before detection. Measurement of the other vessel's bearing on the radar screen is not consistent particularly if the approaching vessel is large, so beware of radar assisted collisions: if the echo of an approaching vessel appears to be on a collision course and it is your duty to keep clear; do so in a positive manner and in ample time.

Navigation by radar

Radar range is accurate but radar bearings can be inconsistent. Steep cliffs and prominent features give a good radar echo at ranges in practice out to 12 miles, but low lying sandbanks and coastal features are frequently not detected outside a range of 3 miles. Many navigation buoys marking primary shipping channels are fitted with radar reflectors which give an enhanced response; but secondary channel buoys may be quite difficult to detect. In rough seas the wave crests cause clutter at close ranges. Radar can 'see' through fog and drizzle but heavy rain showers will be visible on the radar screen and can sometimes obscure shipping or land features.

Radar reflectors

See and be seen. Radar reflectors on small craft enhance the radar return of a radar operating in the vicinity. The degree of enhancement is partly due to the reflecting properties of the elements of the radar reflector but to a greater extent by its size. Whatever the design, a small reflector is unlikely to be as effective as a large one. To a radar, the level of reflection from an object is similar to the reflection of sunlight from a mirror: a concave or flat mirror gives a good reflection provided the angle is right, but a convex mirror scatters the light and the reflection is poor.

A large vessel would expect to detect a motor boat on her radar at a range of about 7 miles. Because her radar is mounted high on the superstructure, the radar may not be able, at ranges of less than 4 miles, to distinguish between the echo received from the boat and sea clutter if there are moderate or rough seas. It is therefore prudent to assume that you have not been detected by a large vessel and to avoid crossing her bows.

Radar Target Enhancers (RTEs)

Radar Target Enhancers are small electronic solid state devices which are fitted as high in the boat as possible. They replace radar reflectors. Whenever they receive the transmitted signal from a radar in the vicinity they will almost instantaneously return an amplified response, thus ensuring that the boat is detected by the radar. They only require a very small amount of current.

These simple devices are completely automatic and require no attention (other than switching them on). More sophisticated versions can produce a warning signal every time they are triggered by a radar transmission.

COMMUNICATION

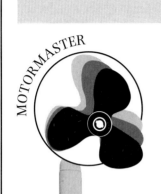

MOTORMASTER

C H A P T E R   S I X T E E N

RADIO

VHF RADIO TELEPHONE

It is advisable for any craft to carry some form of a VHF (very high frequency) radio telephone, (for which a Ship Radio Licence is required, see page 121). This is a radio transmitter/receiver (transceiver) that enables the skipper of a craft to communicate with a coast radio station (connecting to the public exchange network), a port or harbour radio station, and other vessels. In particular a skipper can communicate with the Coastguard and with marinas and yacht harbours; but, most important, can summon assistance in distress or in an emergency. With the exception of the latter instance, any person who uses the radio for transmission must have a Certificate of Competence in Radio Telephony or be directly supervised by such a person. This is because the operation of a radio telephone allows anyone to listen to any transmission; so there has to be a strict discipline controlling any transmissions. It is not difficult to learn and it is in the interest of all skippers to become qualified.

VHF radio communication is essentially a 'line of sight' system and will depend on the antenna heights of the transmitting and receiving station. Between two motor cruisers the effective range is 12 to 15 miles; this could increase to 30 miles between a motor cruiser and a Coast Radio Station with an antenna height of 100 m. The part of the VHF band used for marine communication is from 156 to 163 MHz.

The comparatively short range of VHF radio enables identical frequencies to be used without mutual interference by stations some distance apart. Communication with port services, other ships and marinas is carried out direct from the ship without being routed through a Coast Radio Station. Via a Coast Radio Station a ship or motorboat can be linked to a telephone subscriber almost anywhere in the world.

The various frequencies used in VHF communication are called channels, of which there are some 55 in common use, numbered between 1 and 88. The key channel used for initial calls and distress operations is Channel 16. In United Kingdom waters the Coastguard have special use of Channel 67 for small craft safety traffic.

It is essential that *all* the crew should understand distress and emergency procedures; examples are given in the following section.

A pair of handheld VHF radios and a set (right) which can be surface-mounted. By courtesy of Icom.

Making distress calls

MAYDAY is a distress signal and indicates that a vessel or person is in grave and imminent danger. A distress call has priority over all other traffic. Channel 16 is used for distress and is currently constantly monitored by the Coastguard within United Kingdom waters.

The word MAYDAY is the international distress signal and it is used to alert all boats or shore stations within range that a distress call and message are about to follow. Below are details of how to send such a call together with an example:

Transmitting a distress call

• Check that the main power supply is on.

• Switch the radio to maximum power and tune to channel 16.

• Listen to check that no other station is transmitting.

• Depress the press-to-transmit switch on the microphone.

• Speak clearly and slowly.

The call

1 Repeat MAYDAY three times

2 The words THIS IS

3 The vessel's name or callsign three times

The message

1 MAYDAY once followed by the vessel's name or callsign once.

2 The vessel's position as accurately as possible, either as latitude and longitude or as a true bearing and distance *from* a known geographical point, eg 150° Start Point 2½ miles.

MOTORMASTER

3 The nature of the distress and the assistance required, eg fire, man overboard.

4 The number of persons on board and any other relevant information.

5 The word OVER which means the message is finished and a reply is awaited.

If an immediate reply is not forthcoming, check the operation of the radio and repeat the call at regular intervals.

EXAMPLE

The call

MAYDAY MAYDAY MAYDAY

THIS IS MOTOR VESSEL LINNET, MOTOR VESSEL LINNET, MOTOR VESSEL LINNET

The message

MAYDAY MOTOR VESSEL LINNET

MY POSITION IS TWO ZERO SEVEN DEGREES, LONGSHIPS LIGHTHOUSE FORTY MILES

I AM SINKING AND NEED IMMEDIATE ASSISTANCE

I HAVE FIVE PERSONS ON BOARD

OVER

Urgency

When a very urgent message has to be sent regarding the safety of the vessel or the safety of a person on board, but a MAYDAY signal is not justified, the urgency signal PAN PAN is used. It is transmitted on Channel 16.

The call

1 PAN PAN three times

2 ALL STATIONS, or the name of the station to which the call is addressed, three times

3 The words THIS IS

4 The vessel's name or callsign three times

The message

1 The vessel's position

2 The nature of the urgency and the assistance required

3 The word OVER

EXAMPLE

The call

PAN PAN PAN PAN PAN PAN

ALL STATIONS, ALL STATIONS, ALL STATIONS

THIS IS MOTOR VESSEL PLOVER, MOTOR VESSEL PLOVER, MOTOR VESSEL PLOVER

The message

MY POSITION IS THREE MILES SOUTH OF SAINT CATHERINE'S POINT

ENGINE BROKEN DOWN AND DRIFTING INSHORE

TOW URGENTLY NEEDED

OVER

MOTORMASTER

MEDICAL ADVICE

If medical advice is required the word MEDICO should be included in the urgency call. Use Channel 16 for the initial call and address the call to the nearest Coast Radio Station as you will be connected by telephone to a doctor. After initial acknowledgement you will be requested to change to one of the Coast Radio Station's working channels.

EXAMPLE

PAN PAN   PAN PAN   PAN PAN MEDICO

NORTH FORELAND RADIO, NORTH FORELAND RADIO, NORTH FORE-LAND RADIO

THIS IS MOTOR VESSEL LAPWING, MOTOR VESSEL LAPWING, MOTOR VESSEL LAPWING

MY POSITION IS TWO MILES WEST OF FALLS LIGHT VESSEL

ONE OF MY CREW HAS HAD AN ACCIDENT BREAKING HIS LEG

I REQUIRE MEDICAL ADVICE

OVER

The Coastguard has a VHF radio direction finder and, *in emergencies*, can inform a boat of its position.

SHIP RADIO LICENCE

The Department of Trade and Industry through the Radiocommunications Agency (Ship Radio Licensing Section, Radio-communications Agency, Wray Castle, PO Box 5, Ambleside, LA22 0BF, tel (015394) 34662 administer the issue of a Ship Radio Licence. All vessels with a radio transmitter must hold and display a Ship Radio Licence. When first issued, the licence, which is non transferable between ships, includes the ship's radio call sign, normally four letters and a number, eg MZAB9. Except in emergency a radio operator must hold a Certificate of Competence in Radio Telephony, which is issued following an examination conducted by British Telecom. For small craft with only a short range VHF (Very High Frequency) radio transmitter, a Restricted Certificate of Competence in Radio Telephony (VHF only) is required which is issued following a much simpler test conducted by the Royal Yachting Association. In principle every crew member on a small craft should know how to use the VHF radio transmitter in case of emergency.

MF RADIO TELEPHONE

For radio transmission beyond about 20 miles, a medium frequency single side band (MF SSB) radio transmitter is necessary, operating on the marine band within the frequency range of 1606 to 2850 kHz. The distress and calling frequency is 2182 kHz. (In the USA it is known as the Coastal Harbor Service.) Output power of MF transmitters can vary between 25 watts to 400 watts. The range is affected by the output power, the height of the antenna and weather conditions.

HF RADIO TELEPHONE

If ranges greater than 300 miles are required, the transmitter will have to be capable of working in the high frequency (HF) band. As HF transmission works by bouncing radio waves off the ionosphere where range is dependent on frequency, the Maritime Mobile Service (High Seas

Service in the USA) has slots allocated across the HF band between 3 and 30 MHz. In ideal conditions, ranges greater than 1000 miles may be achieved.

INMARSAT

The global maritime satellite communication system, like the satellite navigation systems, now enables communication to and from ships anywhere in the world. The system is controlled by INMARSAT (International Maritime Satellite Organisation). An INMARSAT subscriber can enjoy direct dialling to over than 100 countries, automatic ship-to-ship calls, telex services, data and facsimile transmission, and immediate connection to the Coastguard Maritime Rescue Co-ordination Centre at Falmouth.

FACSIMILE RECEIVERS

A radio receiver with long wave (148 to 285 kHz) and medium wave (250 to 1606

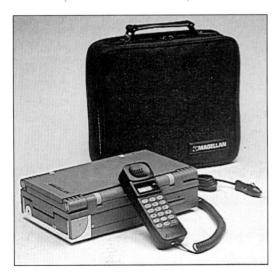

A lap-top satellite telephone will keep you in touch anywhere on the globe. By courtesy of Magellan Systems Corporation.

kHz) bands will receive broadcast weather forecasts and time signals. With special adapters they will receive NAVTEX and WEATHERFAX broadcasts with the latest navigation warnings, shipping forecasts and detailed synoptic (weather) charts.

EMERGENCY POSITION INDICATING RADIO BEACONS

For long distance passage making it is advisable to carry emergency position indicating radio beacons (EPIRBs). When activated these transmit an alarm tone on aircraft distress frequencies which enable the distressed boat or liferaft to be located. As the Global Maritime Distress and Safety System develops, EPIRB transmissions should be received by satellite. The operating frequency used by EPIRBs to communicate with satellites is 406 MHz. If purchasing an EPIRB make sure that it operates on this frequency. The satellite communicating EPIRBs are programmed with a vessel's identity and their position can be fixed worldwide to within 3 miles.

GLOBAL MARITIME DISTRESS AND SAFETY SYSTEM (GMDSS)

GMDSS was devised to provide worldwide distress alert and subsequent communications using INMARSAT satellites with HF as a back up. Provision is made for communication on 2182 kHz and VHF Channel 16. Under the system, distress alerting is either by an EPIRB on 406 MHz or by an automatic push-button system with digital selective calling (DSC) equipment.

Operating procedures are under review, particularly those covering small craft. It is anticipated that a short supplementary qualification to the VHF Restricted Operators Licence may be required.

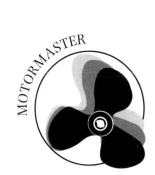

CHAPTER SEVENTEEN

FLAGS

ENSIGNS AND BURGEES

The procedure for flags on ships and boats can appear quite complicated. However here are the basic rules:

- The **national ensign** (an undefaced red ensign for United Kingdom vessels) should be flown at the stern whenever the vessel is at sea and during the day in harbour when a member of the crew is aboard. In harbour the national ensign is hoisted at 0800 in summer and 0900 in winter and lowered at sunset or 2100 whichever is earlier. All times are local times.

- A **club burgee** is flown from a high point on the mast or superstructure at all times when the owner is on board or in control (even though all members of the crew might be temporarily ashore).

- A **courtesy ensign**, a small version of the national ensign of the country visited, should be flown from the starboard side of the superstructure at all times in foreign ports and foreign waters.

Certain countries, the United Kingdom in particular, allow special privilege ensigns to be flown but only if the owner is aboard and is a member of a yacht club which holds a special ensign warrant issued by the Ministry of Defence.

A house flag is the personal flag of the owner or the company association to which the owner belongs. It may be flown from the port side of the superstructure at times when the club burgee is hoisted. The

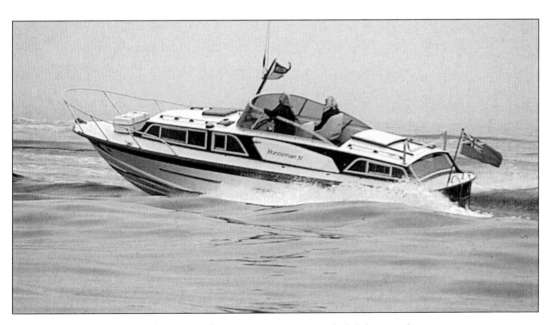

This boat is prominently flying a red ensign at its stern and club burgee from a mast.

Euro flag is regarded as a house flag, not a national ensign. If the owner is not on board or in effective control of the vessel, then his club burgee, house flag and special privilege ensign must not be flown. The standard national ensign and courtesy ensigns shall be flown.

In some countries, various regions have provincial flags. Visitors are encouraged to exhibit these flags, but they should be flown directly below the courtesy ensign.

INTERNATIONAL CODE FLAGS

The International Code Flags together with the International Code Book, enable vessels of any nationality to communicate with each other irrespective of language difficulties. It is unusual for a motor cruiser to carry a full set of flags unless she wishes to dress overall (see below). However, certain flags with single letter meanings should be carried on board. Flag Q, which means 'My vessel is healthy and I request free practique' is used universally as a request for Customs clearance when a vessel is entering a foreign port from another country or returning to her own country from abroad.

Other useful flag meanings are:

Single letters

A   I have a diver down; keep well clear at slow speed.

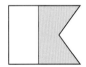

This is one of the most frequently used code flags (blue and white). You will see flown by sport divers on their boats when they are giving cover to divers in the water.

B   I am taking in, or discharging, or carrying dangerous goods.

F   I am disabled; communicate with me.

H   I have a pilot on board.

J   I am on fire and have a dangerous cargo on board: keep well clear of me.

V   I require assistance.

W   I require medical assistance.

Double letters

N over **C**   I am in distress and require immediate assistance.

R over **Y**   You should proceed at alow speed when passing me.

S over **M**   I am undergoing speed trials.

DRESSING SHIP

The ceremonial procedure known as 'Dressing Overall' can take place on three types of occasion: a British national holiday, a foreign festival, a local festival such as a regatta. Ships only dress overall when in harbour or at anchor. The International Code Flags are flown on a line stretching from stem to stern over the mast and superstructure. The order in which they are attached, commencing from the stern, is as follows:

E Q p3 G p8 Z p4 W p6 P p1 I Code T
Y B X 1st H 3rd D F 2nd U A O M R
p2 J p0 N p9 K p7 V p5 L C S

       p = numeral pennant
       Code = code pennant
       1st, 2nd, 3rd = substitute

The order has no particular tradition; it ensures a variety of shape and colour.

USING ROPES AFLOAT

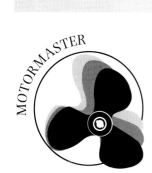

CHAPTER EIGHTEEN

ROPEWORK

Man-made fibre ropes are made of four different types of material:

Nylon This stretches, so it is ideal for anchor or mooring warps.

Polyester (Terylene) This has much less stretch than nylon and is used (particularly in plaited form) for sheets and halyards on yachts.

Polypropylene A buoyant rope which is lightweight, and so it can be used when you want a floating rope to attach to a lifebuoy or as a painter on a dinghy.

Kevlar A strong non-stretching rope. Ropes are supplied either laid up with three strands, plaited or braided. The stranded version is usually laid up right-handed and is coiled in a clockwise direction. Braided or plaited rope twists if coiled the same as laid up rope. It should be coiled in a figure of eight so that the twists cancel out. Ropes are coiled before stowage, for coming alongside and for a heaving line. Stranded ropes can be spliced but braided or plaited ones require special tools and techniques.

All ropes, whether natural or man-made fibre, are subject to chafe. Warps should be protected by passing them through a length of hose, or wrapping a rag around them at the point where they

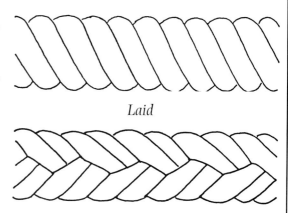

Laid

Plaited

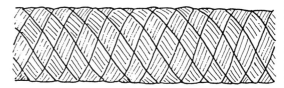

Braided

Ropes can be constructed in several ways: laid by twisting strands together, plaited or braided.

go through the fairlead. Man-made fibres are rot-proof, but should be washed periodically in fresh water to remove any grit or salt which may have worked its way into the rope and can cause damage. They can be damaged by chemicals and heat.

USEFUL KNOTS

Reef knot
Used for joining two ropes of equal size.

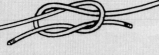

Figure of eight
Used to make a restraining end to a rope ie to prevent a rope pulling out of a block or an eye.

Round turn and two half hitches
A very secure knot for fastening a warp to a mooring ring or pile.

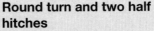
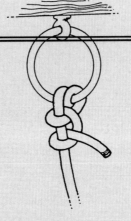

Fisherman's bend
Used for attaching a rope to an anchor. It is not easy to undo after a heavy load has been applied.

Sheet bend
Used to secure a rope's end to an eye or loop, and to attach one rope to another.

Clove hitch
Used to secure a rope to a rail. It isn't a very secure knot as it can slip along a rail and come undone, but it is quick to tie and fine for fastening fenders.

Bowline
A very useful knot. It can be used for making an eye or loop in a rope which will not jam. Handy for slipping over a mooring bollard

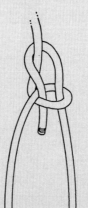
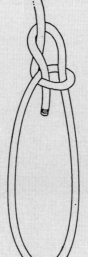

Cleating a rope
A round turn followed by two or three figure of eight turns, finished by a round turn jammed behind the figure of eight turns.

Rolling hitch
A more secure knot for fastening a rope to a spar or another rope under strain when the pull is expected to be from one side.

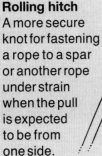

LOAD

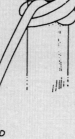

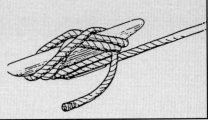

SPLICES & WHIPPING

Back splice

An alternative to a whipping for finishing the end of a rope which is not required to be rove through a block. A crown knot is made (A) and pulled tight (B), and then each strand is tucked over the strand in front of it (C) and under the next one (in the standing part); repeat 3 times.

Eye splice

For making a permanent eye in the end of a rope. In A, strand 1 is tucked under the chosen strand in the standing part. Strand 2 is tucked under the next strand to the left. The splice is then turned over (B). Strand 3 is tucked to the left of strand 2.

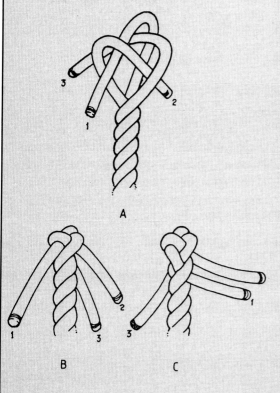

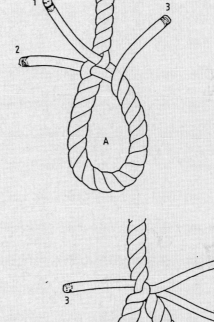

Whipping

Used to tie in the strands at the end of a rope which has been cut.

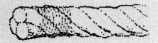

When splicing man-made fibres, the strands of the rope are normally fused using heat. Sticky tape can be used to prevent the rope uncoiling further than intended. A permanent eye splice or back splice may be further protected by a whipping or binding with tape.

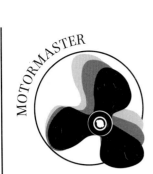
CHAPTER NINETEEN

ANCHORING AND MOORING

Anchoring is a way to prevent the boat from drifting when a temporary stop is necessary. This could be an emergency stop, a short stop for lunch or a longer overnight stay.

Whatever the reason for anchoring, it is essential that the anchor used is of a suitable weight and type to hold the boat in position even under storm conditions. There is always the possibility of engine failure. Should this happen when the boat is near a shore on to which the wind is blowing (a lee shore) the anchor will be the only thing preventing a damaging if not dangerous situation developing.

ANCHORS

There are a variety of anchors available which, at first glance, can be confusing. The four main types are: stock anchor, Danforth anchor, plough anchor and Grapnel. See box feature pages 127–129.

CHOOSING AN ANCHOR

The main consideration when choosing an anchor is its holding power on different types of ground, especially in storm conditions. The only anchor likely to hold well on weed covered rock is the Fisherman anchor. Due to the weight required in comparison with other types and because the stock has to be set by hand, it is less favourable for a main anchor for a motorboat than a Danforth or plough type anchor.

If an electric or electro-hydraulic system is used for lowering and raising the anchor,

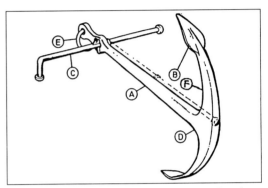

Fig 19.1 *Parts of a stock anchor:* **A** *shank,* **B** *fluke,* **C** *stock,* **E** *ring,* **F** *arm.*

then it is better if the anchor has less moving parts, and the anchor should stow quickly and easily on a bow roller. A Bruce anchor is ideal for this system.

The table on page 130 gives anchor weights and dimensions for different boat lengths. These recommendations, however, are for average boat size and the holding power of an anchor will vary, depending upon the pressure of the wind and the force of the tidal stream or current action upon her hull and superstructure, the shock loads as the boat swings and pitches, the angle at which the cable is pulling, and the quality of the seabed. When purchasing the anchor the storm rather than the working weight should be chosen.

In design terms, fluke area and angle have more significance than weight. Because some anchors are more efficient than others under certain conditions and on differing kinds of seabed, it makes sense to carry on board at least one spare anchor of a different type to the main anchor.

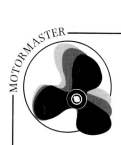

ANCHOR TYPES

FISHERMAN ANCHOR

See Fig 19.1. The Fisherman anchor is also known as a stock anchor. The stock of the anchor, which is collapsible for flatter stowage, is set at right angles to the arms to ensure that the anchor fluke is correctly positioned to dig into the seabed.

Advantages

- Can be stowed flat.

- Good holding power in hard sand and mud and possibly the only type to hold on slippery weed–covered rock.

- Few moving parts to get fouled up and nip fingers.

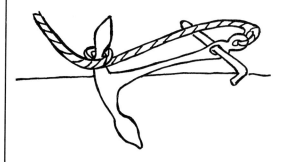

The warp has fouled the fluke of this Fisherman anchor.

Disadvantages

- A Fisherman anchor has to be heavier than other types to give equal holding power.

- When stowed on deck, unless well secured, the flukes can do considerable damage in heavy seas.

- The stock has to be set in position by hand which means that it is not ready for immediate use and is not suitable for an automatic system.

- The fluke, which is vertical above the seabed, can damage the boat if it grounds on it.

- The anchor chain or rope can foul the vertical fluke, or the stock especially as the boat swings on the turn of the tidal stream.

- The retaining pin holding the stock in place can come out, allowing the anchor to collapse and become useless.

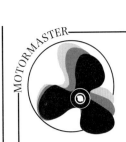

BRUCE ANCHOR

This is a plough type anchor with no movable parts.

Advantages

- It can be lighter than other types and equal their holding power.

- No movable parts to get fouled or trap fingers.

- Digs into the seabed well. As the load is applied, the side fluke digs into the seabed and turns the anchor so that the shank is uppermost. It is so designed that it will be fully embedded within two shank lengths.

- If the wind veers through 90° when it is embedded, it will pivot on the vertical shank without losing its grip or moving more than a few inches.

- With the chain shortened to give a 30° pull on the anchor from the seabed, the anchor will maintain 30% of its holding power and still bury itself. This is useful where there is limited anchorage space or in deeper water.

- Easy to break out.

Disadvantages

- It can only be stowed on deck with a special chock (see photo below). It will not stow flat. However, if well secured it can be stowed over a bow roller.

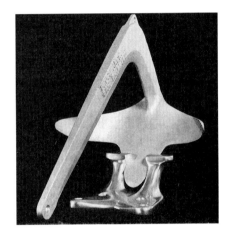

GRAPNEL

A folding grapnel anchor is suitable for dinghies requiring light holding. Grapnels can also be used to lift an obstruction fouling the main anchor.

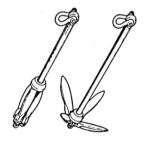

KEDGE ANCHOR

A kedge anchor is any type of small anchor used for a short term anchorage, or possibly for use in conjunction with the main anchor to reduce yawing when in an exposed anchorage.

DANFORTH ANCHOR

Advantages

- Can be stowed flat.
- Less weight is needed to equal the holding power of a Fisherman anchor.
- Good holding power in mud and sand.

Disadvantages

- Movable parts can become fouled or injure fingers.
- Does not hold well in dense weed or rock.
- The anchor falls to the seabed crown first and lies flat. As the strain comes on the anchor the flukes hinge downwards and dig into the bottom. Normally the stronger the pull, the deeper the blades dig in. However, sometimes, when the boat is moving too quickly astern, the flukes may not get a hold and the anchor will drag.
- Can be difficult to break out of mud unless a trip line is used.
- Sometimes it will not dig in on hard sand.

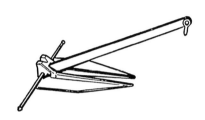

This is a flat, twin fluke anchor with or without a stock across the base of the blades.

CQR ANCHOR

The CQR is a proprietary type of plough-style anchor. The letters are derived from the word 'secure'. The ploughshare shaped blades swivel on a shank so that when the load comes on to the anchor, the tip of the blade digs into the seabed.

Advantages

- Holds well in mud and sand.
- A CQR can be lighter than a Fisherman and still equal its holding power.
- Unless it impales a tin, it digs well in, which makes it more likely to take hold again if it should drag. Filling up the hollow portion with lead improves the holding power even more.

Disadvantages

- It cannot be stowed flat, and so is not really suitable for on deck stowage.
- Movable parts can become fouled and damage the fingers.
- It is cumbersome to handle in a heavy seas.
- It can be difficult to break out unless a tripping line is used.
- Does not hold well in dense weed or on rock.
- Sometimes it will not dig in on hard sand.

SUGGESTED ANCHOR AND CABLE SIZES								
Anchor weight		Maximum boat dimensions		Rode			Anchor shackle	
Storm	Working	Length OA	Beam	Nylon rope dia	Chain dia	Chain weight per m	Pin dia	Body dia
kg	kg	m	m	mm	mm	kg	mm	mm
2	–	5	2.3	10	6	1.13	8	6
5	2	7	2.9	10	6	1.13	8	6
7.5	5	8.5	3.3	10	6	1.13	8	6
10	5	9.8	3.6	14	8	1.40	10	8
15	7.5	12	4.2	16	10	2.20	11	10
20	10	14	4.6	16	10	2.20	11	10
30	15	17.4	5.4	22	13	3.40	16	13
50	20	22	6.3	25	16	3.85	19	16
80	30	27.5	7.0	32	19	7.71	22	19
110	50	32.3	8.1	38	22	10.89	25	22
150	80	38	9.2	44	25	13.88	29	25

ANCHOR CHAIN AND WARP

The anchor is attached to the boat by a cable which consists either of chain or of nylon warp with a short length (6 m) of chain. Before considering which of these choices is best, it is necessary to look at the interaction between anchor and cable.

The holding power of any anchor depends upon a horizontal pull being exerted along the seabed, Fig 19.2. Without this, the anchor will not dig in. This fact is used to advantage when the anchor is broken out before raising. To get this horizontal force sufficient chain or line must be let out when anchoring and the first few metres attached

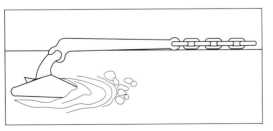

Fig 19.2 *The holding power depends upon the horizontal pull along the sea bed. If there is sufficient weight of chain and length of warp, the anchor will dig in securely.*

to the anchor must have sufficient weight to lie on the seabed.

All chain is the best choice because the weight helps the anchor to work efficiently. Also it is not subject to chafe and it provides a damping action in rough seas. There is, however, one disadvantage – weight. It is impractical for a fast planing boat to carry a large anchor, plus a long length of anchor chain. There is, of course, the problem of recovering it; unless there is a mechanical, electric or electro-hydraulic system available, hauling up a length of anchor chain by hand, with an even heavier anchor attached, can be exhausting.

It is not advisable to use only warp (rope) for anchoring, because the warp has insufficient weight to keep it on the seabed and so will not exert a horizontal pull on the anchor. There is also a problem of chafe on obstructions on the seabed and at any friction points, such as anchor rollers or fairleads (a fitting which guides the direction of the warp).

A good compromise, if weight is a problem, is a combination of chain and warp. At least 6 m of chain should be attached to the anchor; this will have sufficient weight to lie along the seabed and exert a horizontal

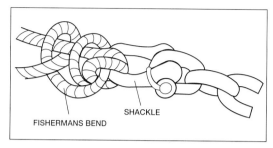

Fig 19.3 *The traditional knot to attach a warp to a chain; make sure you regularly check for chafe.*

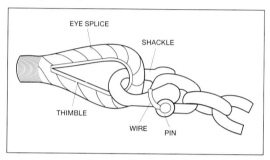

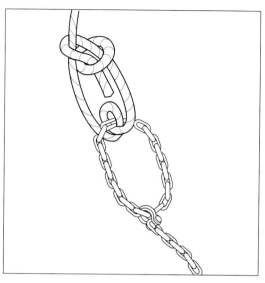

Fig 19.5 *In an emergency you can rig your ground tackle by shackling a loop in the chain and tying the warp to it with a bowline knot.*

Fig 19.4 *Here the anchor chain has been shackled to the warp. To prevent chafe the rope has been spliced round a stainless steel or nylon thimble.*

pull on the anchor. The warp is attached to the other end of this chain. The chain can be attached to the anchor using diameter can be used but you need to watch that it doesn't foul the anchor roller. The warp can be attached to the chain by: a fisherman's bend (Fig 19.3), the warp can be spliced around a thimble to make a loop (called an eye) and a shackle used to join the warp and the chain (Fig 19.4) or the rope can be permanently spliced to the chain. In an emergency, a warp can be joined to a chain by shackling a loop in the chain, passing the warp through this loop, turning it once around the chain and then securing by tying a bowline (Fig 19.5).

When shackles are used, a wire must be rove (passed) through the shackle pin and twisted around the shackle to prevent the pin turning.

The inboard end of the chain or warp should be secured so that it can easily be released in an emergency. Usually it is secured with a light line that can easily be cut. This line should not be relied upon to hold the chain or warp when anchored, and the load should be taken by turning around a cleat. When a windlass is fitted, there is a braking system for this purpose.

For assessing the length of chain to be let out the following rules apply:

Chain only	Four times the maximum water depth.
Chain and warp	Six times the maximum water depth.
Strong tidal stream and/or strong wind	Eight times the maximum water depth.

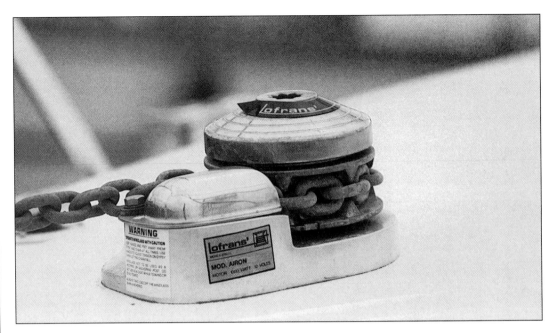

This Lofrans all-chain electric windlass can be operated from the cockpit.

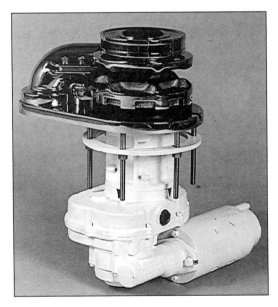

Expanded view of chain/rope windlass showing power drive.

Windlasses

To help with handling the anchor, a windlass can be fitted on the boat. This can be operated manually, or electrically using a foot switch on the foredeck, or the whole operation can be carried out without leaving the wheelhouse.

It is better to have all chain anchoring systems, especially if using an electrical system, although there are several models that will deal with chain or warp, (see photos). The diameter of chain used should be suitable for the anchor size and the windlass. (A guide to chain diameters is given in the table on page 130).

Anchor chain or warp should be marked at various intervals along its length so that you know at a glance how much you have let out.

Anchor stowage

The main anchor must be ready for immediate use, with its chain shackled on. This means that it has to be stowed in, on or over the bows. It must also be secured so there is no possibility of its breaking loose and causing damage when the boat is underway.

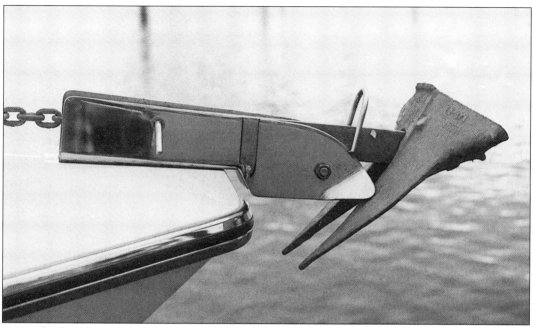

A Danforth type anchor mounted on the bow. The safety pin secures it in position. For operation, the pin is removed and the anchor can be lowered or raised remotely from the cockpit.

Secured on deck

The anchor can be secured on deck and kept in place by chocks. The chain is led through a pipe into a locker below the deck. The disadvantage of this is that it has to be unchocked and manoeuvred into position manually when needed. It is also liable to cause an accident to anyone falling on it or over it.

Stowed in anchor locker

This is slightly better than deck stowage. However there is still the problem of lifting the anchor manually into position for lowering. If the locker is the type with a hinged lid, this can in itself be a hazard in rough weather should someone fall on the lid or into the locker. The anchor and chain must be secured inside the locker so that there is no movement underway. Locker stowage does have the advantage of keeping the deck clear.

Over the bow stowage

This is the best system for easy access and immediate use. The anchor is secured over a bow roller, and the chain led back directly to an anchor locker or to an anchor locker via a windlass. It is the only suitable stowage when an electrical windlass is used. When the anchor is raised, the chain followed by the shank is pulled over a bow roller, or rollers into its stowage position. Chain tension between the anchor and the windlass keeps it in place. It may be necessary to fit an additional pin through the anchor shank to stop lateral and vertical movement which can occur in heavy seas, (See photo above.)

Secondary anchor stowage

Additional anchors should be stowed securely in a readily accessible place.

MOTORMASTER

CHOOSING AN ANCHORAGE

When selecting an anchorage, you should first check the wind direction and strength for present and expected winds. It is worth considering the general trend and the local forecast. Weather information is dealt with in Chapter 20. An anchorage may appear inviting, especially after a tiring passage, but if anything but a short stay is intended, consider what the situation is likely to be several hours later, to avoid having to move the boat in the middle of the night.

You also need to think about the effects of the tidal stream throughout your stay. Ideally, the chosen position should be out of the area where the tidal stream flows strongest. In a bay, the tidal stream tends to flow less strongly nearer to the shore, but not always in the same direction as the main tidal stream. This is a point to bear in mind when approaching the anchorage position. A pilot book gives information about specific anchorages and will have general information about tidal streams, but as there are local peculiarities, it is generally only a guide. Anchorages are marked on some charts by an anchor symbol.

The topography of the coastline is also important. By day, a bay surrounded by a high cliffy coastline or in the proximity of mountains, may be very sheltered. However, as night approaches and the land cools, air next to the land also cools, becomes heavier and rolls seawards causing an offshore breeze. Depending on the gradient and height of the coastline, quite strong winds can build up overnight, especially where there are gaps in the cliffs which may cause funnelling.

It is important to be able to leave an anchorage at any time, day or night, in any wind direction or in poor visibility. Day transits or lights by night are a useful guide but if the anchorage cannot be negotiated without using these, a careful watch must be kept on visibility.

Other considerations are:

- Good holding ground; no obstructions.

- Clear of obstructions and other boats throughout the full swinging circle of the boat. Boats with different keels do not all lie in the same direction in an anchorage.

- A position where there is sufficient water for the duration of the stay.

- A position where the boat has enough chain or warp for the maximum depth and for all weather conditions. This means, at least 4 times the maximum depth if chain is used, and 6 times if warp is used. If there is a lot of wave action lifting the bows then more chain or warp should be let out. When bad weather is expected, use at least 8 times the maximum depth of chain or warp.

- Stay out of areas used frequently by other boats.

- If going ashore, moor near a suitable landing stage.

- Stay away from areas where other boats are moored to buoys, as the anchor can foul the ground tackle to which these buoys are secured.

There should be a suitable back-up plan. If possible an alternative anchorage should be available, preferable downwind. Don't forget to switch on your anchor light at night.

Lowering the anchor

When the anchorage is reached put the engines into neutral; as the boat ceases forward movement, release the anchor to the seabed. Let out sufficient chain or warp and make sure that the inboard end is secured to the boat! It may be necessary to run the engines in reverse to help the anchor to dig in. Look for some landmarks to use as transits to check that the anchor is not dragging. If it is dragging, then let out more chain or warp, or raise the anchor and look for a better location.

Trip line

If you think that there may be obstructions on the seabed and there is no other suitable position in which to anchor, then use a trip line. A trip line is a light line secured at one end to the crown of the anchor and at the other end to a small buoy. You use this line to pull the anchor out by the flukes if it becomes fouled on an obstruction (Fig 19.6).

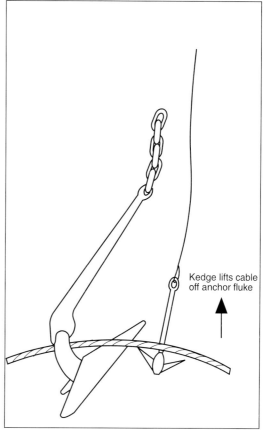

Kedge lifts cable off anchor fluke

Fig 19.7 *A main anchor caught under a cable may be freed by dropping the second anchor (kedge) which can lift the cable sufficiently to release the anchor.*

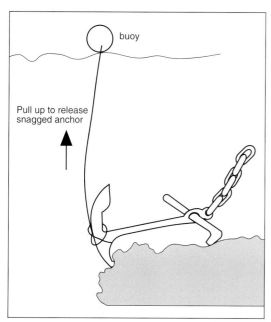

buoy

Pull up to release snagged anchor

Fig 19.6 *If you think your anchor may get snagged, rig a trip line as shown here.*

Fouled Anchor

If your anchor becomes fouled upon an obstruction and you haven't fitted a trip line, you may lose anchor and some chain. If there is a chance of recovering it later, then attach a buoy. It may be possible to drag it free by motoring in the direction opposite to that in which the anchor was laid. The kedge anchor can be used to lift the obstruction, especially if this is a cable (Fig 19.7). This may result in the loss of the kedge but it is preferable to losing the main anchor and chain.

MOTORMASTER

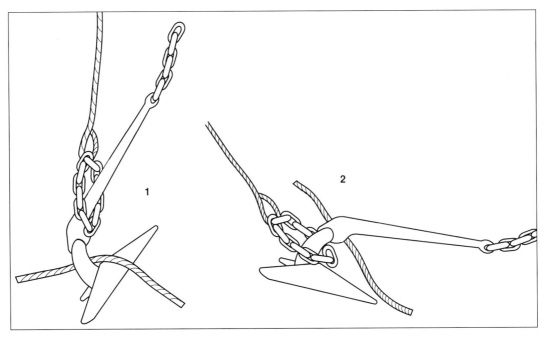

Fig 19.8 *Freeing a fouled anchor with a chain.*

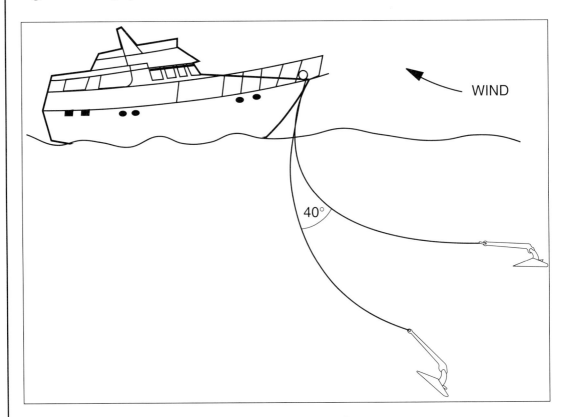

Fig 19.9 *Using a second anchor when the boat is wind-rode.*

Alternatively, the following method can be tried (Fig 19.8):

1 Haul in the chain until it is vertical.

2 Attach a line to a heavy object such as a large shackle or several loops (a clump) of chain and lower it around the anchor chain down to the anchor.

3 Buoy the anchor chain and lower overboard.

4 The line attached to the clump of chain is secured to a strong stern cleat and the boat motored away in the direction opposite to which the anchor was laid. The lower point of purchase on the anchor may drag it clear.

Using a second anchor

You may need to use a second anchor to stop the boat yawing (swinging from side to side) in a strong wind, or to limit the swinging circle due to the tidal stream.

When the boat is wind-rode (head to wind) and there are no effects from the tidal stream, lead both anchors from the bows with an angle of about 40° between them (Fig 19.9).

If you need to limit the swinging circle where there is a strong tidal stream, lay both anchors from the bows but in the direction of the tidal stream. Lay the heaviest anchor into the strongest tidal stream (Fig 19.10). This method is not suitable if there is a strong cross wind as both anchors will drag.

Warning: Anchoring fore and aft is not suitable for a small boat as too great a strain is put on the boat. Also, both anchors may drag in a strong cross wind or tidal stream.

MOORING TECHNIQUES

Terms used for mooring:

Bow line A rope from the bows of the boat leading forward.

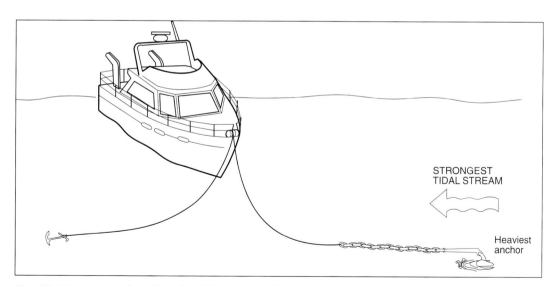

Fig 19.10 *A second anchor should be used if there is a strong tidal stream. Make sure that you have at least 6–10 metres of chain between anchor and warp to give a good horizontal pull on the anchor.*

MOTORMASTER

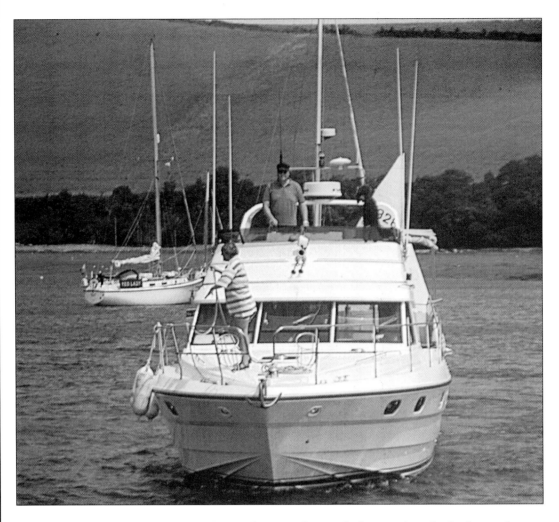

This cruiser is approaching her berth at a slow, steady speed; the crew has the fenders and ropes ready to moor.

Breast ropes Ropes abreast of the boat from the bows and stern. These are particularly useful for coming into a berth. They should be slightly slack.

Springs Diagonal ropes from the bows leading aft and from the stern leading forward. These stop the boat moving fore and aft and should be taut.

Stern line A rope from the stern of the boat leading aft.

Bollard, **cleat** or **bitt** Names of fittings on the boat or ashore to which mooring lines can be secured.

Snubber A strong spring or section of rubber which absorbs the tug on mooring lines due to wind, waves or boat's wash.

Pontoon a structure of planks which form a catwalk or platform alongside to which boats can be moored.

Pile Wooden, concrete or metal posts driven into the sea or river bed.

MOTORMASTER

Mooring alongside

Mooring a motorboat alongside a harbour wall or pontoon is not really very difficult once you are familiar with your boat. Your boat should have good manoeuvrability especially if you have twin engines and a bow thruster (a prop fitted at the bow to push it to port or starboard as required). Like most skills, mooring needs practice, some forward planning and a good briefing for the crew.

Bear in mind that it is usually easier to approach a berth into the tidal stream but you should check the wind direction because you will have a more comfortable night if you are moored head to wind. Have your crew ready to jump ashore with ropes and make sure that there are sufficient fenders down on the correct side. The configuration of mooring lines that are suitable for lying alongside are shown in Fig 19.11. In a marina or in a berth where there is a very small rise and fall of tide, the bow and stern lines need not be so long.

Sometimes it is necessary to tie up to another boat which may be part of a 'raft' of boats. Try to select a boat of similar size and freeboard height as your own. If there is someone aboard the adjacent boat, out of courtesy ask permission to lie alongside and cross over their decks. The classic response from a yacht skipper is 'Yes, fine, but I'm catching the tide at 4 am!'

You will need breast and spring ropes secured to the next boat but you *must* attach bow and stern lines to points ashore. If you don't, you may find yourself adrift at 0410!

If you arrive at night, be very considerate to the occupants of the boat you are next to, especially if you are going ashore and have to walk across their boat. This especially applies when you return after a good dinner ashore!

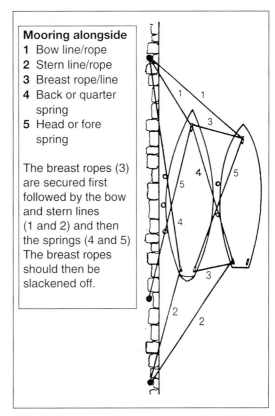

Mooring alongside
1 Bow line/rope
2 Stern line/rope
3 Breast rope/line
4 Back or quarter spring
5 Head or fore spring

The breast ropes (3) are secured first followed by the bow and stern lines (1 and 2) and then the springs (4 and 5) The breast ropes should then be slackened off.

Fig 19.11   *Mooring alongside. Any lines taken ashore must be adjusted as the tide rises or falls. Thus the outside boat must adjust her bow and stern lines, whilst her springs and breast ropes, which are taken to the inside boat, need not be adjusted.*

Picking up a buoy

In a strong tidal stream, always approach the mooring with your bow into the tidal stream, allowing for windage if there is a strong wind. You may have problems if the wind is against the tide.

Ideally, you should have two crew members on the bow: one to catch the buoy with a boathook and the other to secure a strong line to it. Some mooring buoys have a line with a small buoy attached to the main line which is easier to pick up. Once you have secured your line to the buoy you could fasten your anchor chain to the buoy for extra security.

Mooring between two piles

Any craft moored between two piles must have her own bow and stern lines fastened to the piles – do not rely on someone else's lines. If the mooring is empty, approach the piles into the tidal stream. Try to get a line from the bow through the mooring ring on the upstream pile then drop back to repeat the manoeuvre with the stern to the down-stream pile. Balance the boat's position by hauling in or easing off the bow and stern lines. If the lines are looped (doubled back) through the mooring rings, it is much easi-er to depart when necessary.

If another boat is already on the moor-ing, then go alongside that craft (see Mooring alongside), preferable pointing in the same direction. When secure, bow and stern lines can be rigged using the dinghy.

If you are leaving the boat for several days, the lines can become chafed on the mooring rings and on the boat's fairleads. Wrap cloth or rubber tubing around the lines to prevent chafing.

Mediterranean mooring

In the Mediterranean and other places where there is little rise and fall of tide, it is customary to moor with the bow or stern close to the quayside with the other end of

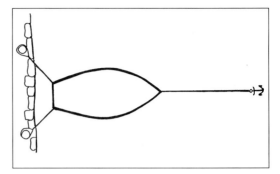

Fig 19.12 *Mediterranean mooring.*

the boat secured to a buoy or anchored.

In established marinas there is often a light line dropping into the water from the quayside which, when hauled in, will be attached to a mooring line on an offshore anchorage. Having gently manoeuvred the boat so her bow or stern are ready on the quayside, a line can be taken to a strong point (bollard) ashore and the mooring line can be hauled in and secured at the sea-ward end. It is normally the practice (see Fig 19.12) to have two lines secured ashore to prevent lateral movement. It is better seamanship to moor with the stern alongside and the bow facing to seaward.

It is more difficult to manoeuvre if a line has to be secured to a buoy or if it is neces-sary to drop an anchor before attaching the shore line. However, with practice it can be done speedily and efficiently.

QUESTIONS

19.1 What is a trip line and when should it be used?

19.2 What length of anchor chain should be let out in calm conditions for a maximum depth of 4 m?

19.3 How would you ensure that the anchor is not dragging?

19.4 What would be your considerations for choosing an anchorage?

19.5 When should a second anchor be used?

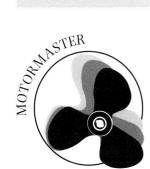

CHAPTER TWENTY

WEATHER SYSTEMS

What is the weather going to do? For the seafarer, information about what the weather is doing, and more important what it is likely to do, is vital not only to ensure a comfortable passage but also a safe one. The two main hazards on open water are strong winds, which create waves, and any condition, such as fog, which impairs visibility.

WIND

Too little wind is not a problem as far as a power vessel is concerned. Too much wind, however, can make manoeuvring within the harbour difficult and in open water lead to an uncomfortable if not dangerous passage. A strong wind creates waves which can force the boat to reduce speed considerably. If a planing boat is forced to reduce speed to displacement mode, it can lead to an uncomfortable situation. Such a boat is designed to motor with most of its hull clear of the water, so its hull shape will make it difficult to handle in heavy weather at slow speeds.

Sea breezes

On a warm sunny day the land heats up relatively quickly. Air in contact with the land is heated and rises, drawing in cooler air from the sea creating a sea breeze. This

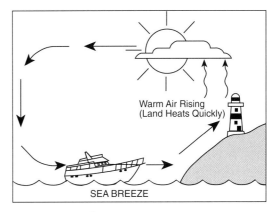

Fig 20.1 *Sea breeze.*

generally starts about late morning, strengthens during the afternoon and dies out by sunset, Fig 20.1. Sea breezes can reach force 4 (see Beaufort Scale in Chapter 21) and be felt some five miles offshore. They are more noticeable in settled weather conditions, but are masked by strong winds. When sea breezes are prevalent, a power driven craft may find calmer water offshore.

Land breeze

After sunset, especially if there is a clear sky, the land loses heat by radiation. Air in contact with the land is cooled, becomes heavier and rolls out to sea. The land breeze persists between around midnight and dawn, Fig 20.2. Generally on the same

141

MOTORMASTER

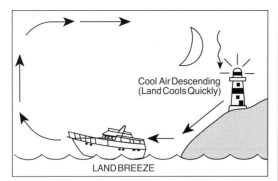

Fig 20.2 *Land breeze.*

day in the same area the land breeze is lighter than the sea breeze.

Anabatic wind

This occurs during the day due to surface heating of a sloping surface such as a mountain side, particularly one facing the sun. Air heated by contact with the land rises and flows up the mountain.

Katabatic wind

This is similar to a land breeze and occurs at night on sloping ground. As the land cools, air in contact with it cools and rolls down the slope. In mountainous areas a strong wind develops which is further increased if it funnels along a valley to seaward. A boat anchored overnight in the vicinity of mountains may experience very uncomfortable conditions after dark as the strong wind blows down the slope and out to sea.

Wave heights

The height of a wave is principally determined by wind strength but the following factors also play a part.

Fetch

With an offshore wind, the distance trav-

Mediterranean winds

In the Mediterranean there are many local winds some of which are shown in Fig 20.3. In northern summer the permanent high pressure system over the Azores influences the western Mediterranean whilst the eastern Mediterranean is affected by low pressure over the Asian land mass (which is also responsible for monsoons in the Indian Ocean).

Mistral

A strong north or northwest wind which is cold and dry giving generally sunny clear weather. As it can reach force 8 or more, especially in winter when it is re-inforced by the katabatic winds from the Alps funnelling along the Rhône valley, rough sea conditions can ensue.

Tramontana

This is a cold dry north or northeast wind associated with winter depressions. It blows on to Corsica from the west coast of Italy in winter but is not often gale force. It is associated with a depression over the Adriatic and is an extension of the mistral.

Vendevales

A strong southwesterly wind blowing into the Straits of Gibraltar, associated with depressions especially during winter months. It funnels through the Straits increasing in strength.

Scirocco or Leveche

A hot dry dust-laden wind from the south originating in the North African desert. It

elled by the wind between shore and boat is called the fetch. Wave height increases with fetch so a boat further offshore will experience rougher conditions.

Duration of blow

The length of time the wind has been blowing in a given direction also affects wave

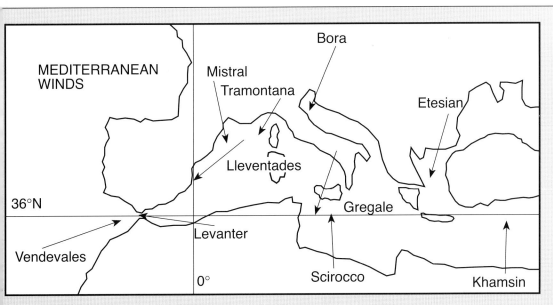

Fig 20.3 *Mediterranean winds.*

becomes moisture laden as it crosses the sea and arrives on northern shores warm and humid often causing fog.

Levanter
A moist easterly wind which funnels through the Straits of Gibraltar causing bad visibility, cloud and rain. Associated with high pressure over western Europe and low pressure to the southwest of Gibraltar.

Gregale
A strong northeast wind which affects the western and central Mediterranean. North facing harbours in Malta and Sicily are particularly exposed. It occurs when there is high pressure to the north and low pressure to the south.

Etesians or Melterni
A fresh northerly wind giving fine clear weather in summer.

Khamsin
A dust-carrying southerly wind in the eastern Mediterranean in front of a depression. Similar to the Scirocco.

Bora
A strong north to easterly katabatic wind which is cold and dry from the Adriatic. It occurs mainly in winter sometimes behind a depression.

height. Initially waves may be short and steep but as the wind continues they increase in height and become longer. Should the wind change direction, say, from a fresh southwesterly to a strong northwesterly, the established southwesterly wave pattern will persist for a while but a new wave pattern caused by the northwesterly wind will be superimposed upon it. This will cause a confused sea until the effect of the southwesterly wave pattern dies away.

Shallow water
When the wind is blowing towards the shore (a leeshore) waves travelling over a shoaling seabed become shorter and

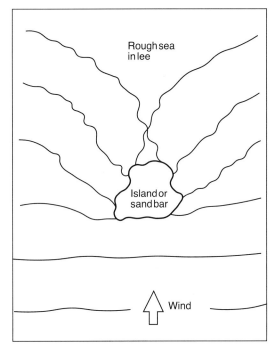

Fig 20.4 *Cross waves.*

increase in height eventually breaking and causing surf. In a strong wind situation a leeshore is a dangerous place to be.

Tidal stream

When the wind is blowing against the flow of the tidal stream, waves can break causing unpleasant and sometimes hazardous conditions. This is worst with a strong wind against a spring tide. When the wind is blowing in the same direction as the tidal flow, the water surface will be flatter. It may be possible to make a passage under these conditions which would not have been feasible with wind against tide.

Tidal race

If there is an uneven rocky ledge extending out from a headland, projecting into the main tidal stream, the water races around the headland causing whirlpools known as overfalls. A boat caught in these overfalls in strong winds would be tossed about and

find steering difficult. Tidal races are strongest at spring tides.

Sometimes there is an inshore passage close to land clear of the race, but this should not be attempted without careful planning and a knowledge of the area as timing can be critical. It is generally safer to pass to seaward of a race, which may be ten nautical miles or so offshore.

Reflected waves

Waves pounding a harbour wall or breakwater in relatively deep water will be reflected back and interact with more incoming waves causing steep confused seas. This may make entry to such a harbour difficult or dangerous.

Cross waves

Waves hitting the weather side of a shoal or island can be deflected around, converging on the lee side and causing rough seas. A boat seeking a sheltered anchorage in the lee of an island could find an uncomfortable sea, Fig 20.4.

Funnelling

Wind blowing through a narrow channel, for example between an island and a headland, speeds up as it funnels through the bottleneck, fanning out at the lee end of the channel. The worst sea conditions will occur when the wind direction is in opposition to a spring tidal stream.

Swell

Swell is wind generated waves which have travelled a long distance away from where they were formed. It can be present on an otherwise calm day and may be a warning of approaching bad weather.

VISIBILITY

Conditions which affect visibility are: smoke and dust causing haze, and precipitation such as rain, hail, snow, mist and fog.

Fog

Air can hold moisture in the form of water vapour in direct proportion to its temperature. The warmer the air, the more moisture it can hold. When air is holding all the moisture it can for a given temperature it is saturated and is said to have reached its dew point. If it is cooled below dew point condensation occurs and if conditions are favourable fog forms.

Cooling

Cooling can be caused by:

* The proximity of cold land.

* A cold sea surface.

* Two adjacent air masses of different temperatures both of which are near saturation level.

Radiation fog

Radiation fog is caused by land cooling at night. It forms over land but can drift out to sea for several miles obscuring the coastline. It occurs when the land cools after a relatively warm day, especially if there is a clear night sky when much heat is lost by radiation (see Fig 20.5).

If air in contact with the land is cooled below its dew point condensation occurs and, if conditions are right, this will form fog. Conditions necessary for the formation of radiation fog are:

* Moisture laden air especially at low level.

* Clear sky.

* A little wind at surface level to create turbulent mixing. Too much wind will result in low cloud, too little in marsh mist forming a few centimetres above the ground.

* A cold wet land surface.

* A relatively long cold night such as in autumn or winter.

Radiation fog is often most dense about an hour after sunrise when the land temperature is still low and the heat from the sun causes slight turbulence. It usually disperses at midday when solar heating is

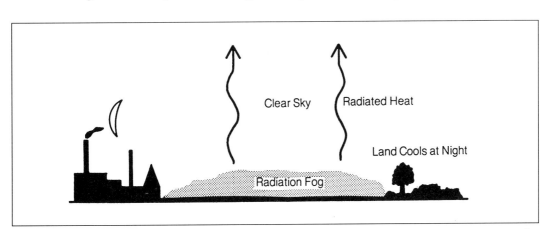

Fig 20.5 *Radiation fog forming at night. This forms over land, but can then drift out to sea for several miles.*

strongest; but sometimes, in the winter, it can persist all day.

Advection fog

Advection or sea fog occurs when a warm damp air mass moves over a progressively colder sea surface; it can also form over land. The fog forms when the air is cooled below its dew point. Sea fog can persist in winds up to force 6. An example of this is a moist southwesterly air stream moving into the English Channel especially in spring and early summer when the sea is at its coldest. It may disperse when a change of wind direction brings drier air.

Frontal fog

Frontal fog occurs along the boundary of two air masses with very different characteristics when both air masses are near saturation point, such as warm or cold fronts.

Action in deteriorating visibility

Although visibility may be good at the start of a passage, it can deteriorate later, sometimes unexpectedly. Perhaps the horizon becomes indistinct, or vessels which were clearly visible seem to have disappeared. Maybe the sun does not seem as bright as it did. Ahead, in the distance, a fog bank may be visible.

The action to take in these circumstances depends upon the boat's position, other shipping and navigational hazards around the boat, the availability of electronic equipment and the experience of the navigator. The following points are a guide:

1   Slow down and obtain a fix of position. Record the time, log reading and, if appropriate, depth. If it is not possible when out of sight of land to obtain a fix, then the estimated position must be carefully worked out.

2   Observe the position of any other shipping in the area.

3   Refer to the chart to see if there are likely to be any navigational hazards on the intended track which may be difficult to negotiate in fog. If this is the case, then an alternative destination with easy access should be considered. This may mean returning to the port of origin or seeking a safe anchorage.

4   If in a Traffic Separation Scheme, clear it as soon as possible but keep the boat's course at right angles to the direction of the traffic flow.

5   Reduce the boat's speed sufficiently to enable it to stop in good time in an emergency to avoid a collision or grounding.

6   Switch on and use all available electronic equipment for position finding and collision avoidance.

7   If not permanently fitted, hoist the radar reflector or activate the radar target enhancer..

8   Put on lifejackets and make sure the liferaft is in a position where it can be launched quickly if needed.

9   Sound the appropriate fog signal (one prolonged blast at intervals not exceeding two minutes).

10 Post a bow lookout to listen as well as watch. Maintain silence.

11 If following a buoyed channel, make a list of the buoys with their characteristics and the direction and distance from one buoy to the next. Mark off the buoys as they are passed, comparing the distance and elapsed time between them. Use the echo-sounder to keep within the channel and remember to which side of the boat the safe water

lies. Listen for other shipping in the channel. In a busy commercial harbour, if there is sufficient water, navigate just outside the main buoyed channel but still within sight of the buoys.

12 When approaching a harbour clear of offlying dangers, it is good strategy to set a course to one side of the entrance so that when the shoreline is sighted or a particular depth contour reached, there is no doubt which way to alter course for the harbour entrance. If the course is well upstream the tidal stream will be fair on the approach to the entrance.

13 Listen for the fog signals of lighthouses. It is not easy to determine the direction of sounds in foggy conditions. If there is a marine radiobeacon at the harbour entrance, the Radio Direction Finder can be used to keep it on a constant bearing in order to locate the harbour entrance.

HOW WEATHER SYSTEMS DEVELOP

The earth's surface is heated by solar radiation. However, the heating is not uniform. The same amount of heat is spread over a wider area at the Poles than at the Equator, so it is hotter at the Equator than at the Poles. Rising and descending air, caused by varying surface temperatures and assisted by the earth's rotation, cause permanent and semi-permanent pressure systems to develop. Pressure on the surface of the earth is low in areas where hot air is rising and high where cold air is descending.

Large land masses cool and heat quicker than adjacent sea areas, causing high pressure in winter and low pressure in summer. Global pressure distribution for January and July is shown in Figs 20.6 and 20.7.

Low pressure systems

In a low pressure system, air rising at the centre causes surrounding air at surface

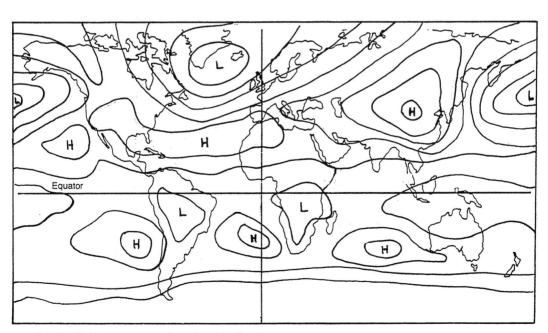

Fig 20.6 Global pressure distribution for January.

MOTORMASTER

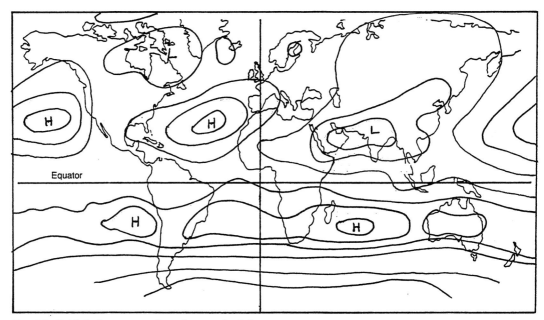

Fig 20.7 *Global pressure distribution for July.*

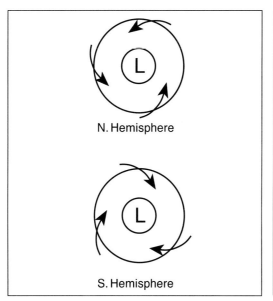
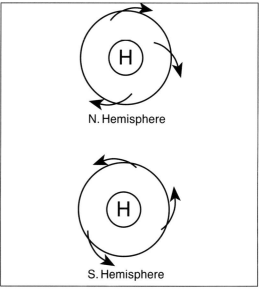

Figs 20.8 and 20.9 *Left: A low pressure system: air moves in an anti-clockwise direction in N hemisphere..*
Right: A high pressure system or anti-cyclone: Air moves in a clockwise direction in N hemisphere.

level to flow inwards. Due to the rotational effect of the earth, the air does not follow a direct path but spirals around the centre resulting in an anti-clockwise circulation in the northern hemisphere and a clockwise circulation in the southern hemisphere. The lowest pressure is at the centre of the system, Fig 20.8.

High pressure systems

In a high pressure system, air descends at the centre and flows outwards at surface level following a spiral pattern. In the northern hemisphere the circulation is clockwise, whilst in the southern hemisphere it is anti-clockwise. The highest pressure will be at the centre of the system, Fig 20.9.

Air masses

Air is constantly moving from areas of higher pressure to areas where the pressure is lower. Its characteristics will initially be that of its source region, but as it moves over the earth's surface it becomes modified by the areas over which it travels. Air from arctic and polar regions will be cold, whilst that from tropical or equatorial regions will be warm.

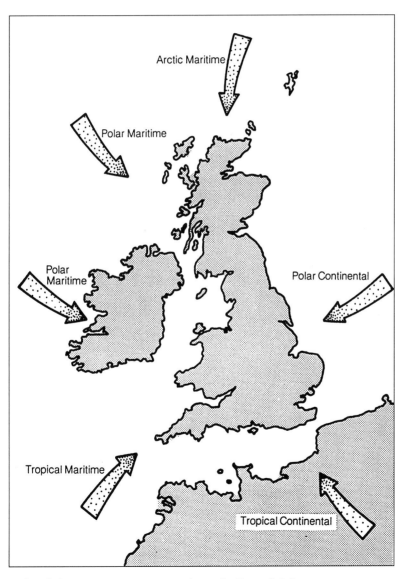

Fig 20.10 *Tracks of the main air masses reaching the British Isles.*

WEATHER ASSOCIATED WITH A DEPRESSION

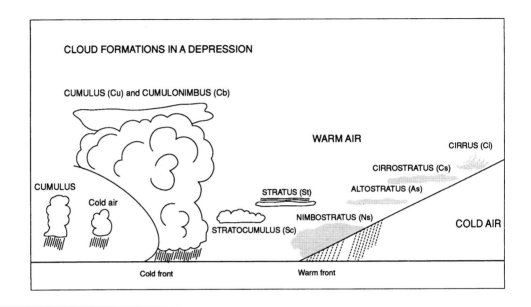

CLOUD FORMATIONS IN A DEPRESSION

CUMULUS (Cu) and CUMULONIMBUS (Cb)

WARM AIR

CIRRUS (Ci)

CIRROSTRATUS (Cs)

CUMULUS

Cold air

ALTOSTRATUS (As)

STRATUS (St)

NIMBOSTRATUS (Ns)

COLD AIR

STRATOCUMULUS (Sc)

Cold front   Warm front

	Before warm front	On warm front	Warm sector	On cold front	After cold front
Cloud (in order of appearance)	Ci Cs As Ns	Ns	St Sc Cu Cb	Cu Cb	As Ac Cu Cb blue sky
Precipitation	Continuous rain, light at first, becoming moderate	Rain turning to drizzle	Drizzle or intermittent slight rain, possible fog, heavy rain near cold front	Heavy rain, snow, hail; maybe thunder	Continuous heavy rain giving way to heavy showers
Visibility	Good at first deteriorating in rain	Poor maybe mist or fog	Moderate to poor, mist or fog	Poor in heavy rain	Improves rapidly to very good except in showers
Barometer	Falls steadily	Steadies	Little change	Sudden rise	Rapid continuous rise becoming slower later
Wind	Freshens	Veers	Steady	Sudden veer, strengthens, squally	Steady in direction, strong at first decreasing later

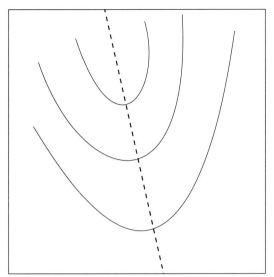

Fig 20.11 *Trough.*

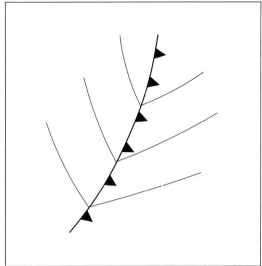

Fig 20.12 *Frontal trough.*

The main air masses affecting the British Isles are shown in Fig 20.10. Their characteristics are:

Polar Continental (Pc)
Cold and dry, bringing very cold and often cloudy weather especially in winter. Source region: the Siberian high pressure zone.

Arctic Maritime and Polar Maritime (Am, Pm)
Very cold and moist, associated with cumulus and cumulonimbus cloud, squally showers and hail. Source region: the Polar and arctic high pressure zones.

Tropical Maritime (Tm)
Warm and moist bringing cloud, rain, drizzle and fog or generally poor visibility. Source region: Azores high pressure zone.

Tropical Continental (Tc)
Warm and dry giving clear sky but possibly haze. Source region: North Africa, Southern Europe.

Trough of low pressure

A trough of low pressure is an extension of a low pressure system where the isobars form a U or V shape away from the lowest pressure, Fig 20.11. When a front is present it is called a frontal trough, Fig 20.12.

Tropical revolving storm

In late summer in tropical regions between latitudes 3° and 10° north and south, a Tropical Revolving Storm (TRS) may form. These travel at a rate of about 10 knots in a westerly direction across the oceans moving gradually away from the Equator. They are associated with very strong winds and high seas. When making a passage in these areas, it is wise to monitor the local weather stations to ascertain the likelihood of such a storm occurring.

Anti-cyclone

An anti-cyclone is a high pressure system (see Fig 20.9).

MOTORMASTER

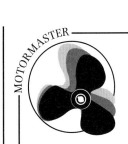

WEATHER FRONTS

When two air masses with different characteristics meet, they do not mix readily. The boundary between them is called a front. The Polar Front separates polar air from tropical air. Other fronts are: the Mediterranean Front which separates cold winter air over Europe and warm air over North Africa; the Inter Tropical Convergence Zone (ITCZ) which is between the Trade Wind belts and the Doldrums. The Doldrums are a windless area extending up to 10° either side of the Equator with the Trade Wind belts (steady winds) another 10° on either side.

HOW A FRONTAL DEPRESSION FORMS

A A frontal depression in temperate latitudes is a low pressure system which forms along the Polar Front. It starts as a wave along the surface of the Polar Front. The rising air from the warm air mass causes a pressure drop at the tip of the wave.

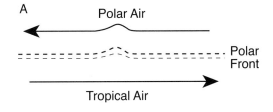

B The wave develops and there is a further fall in pressure. The system continues to develop distorting the Polar Front.

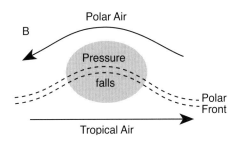

C Pressure falls further in the middle as air rises. A cyclonic circulation develops around the point of lowest pressure, and the Polar Front is now distorted to an inverted V shape. For ease of reference the leading edge of the warmer wedge of air is referred to as the *warm front* and the leading edge of the colder air as the *cold front*. The lines shown are *isobars*, contour lines of equal pressure.

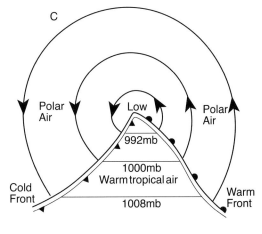

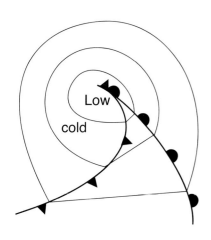

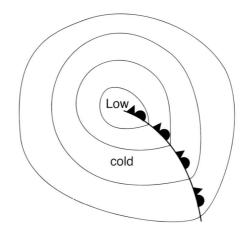

D The cold front gradually overtakes the warm front, a process which is known as an *occlusion*.

E Eventually the warm front is completely overtaken and the depression is fully occluded. After occluding, the depression slows down and starts to fill.

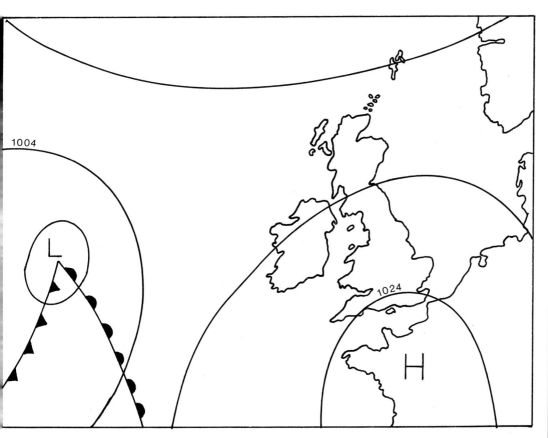

A simplified version of how weather fronts are given on a meteorological synoptic chart.

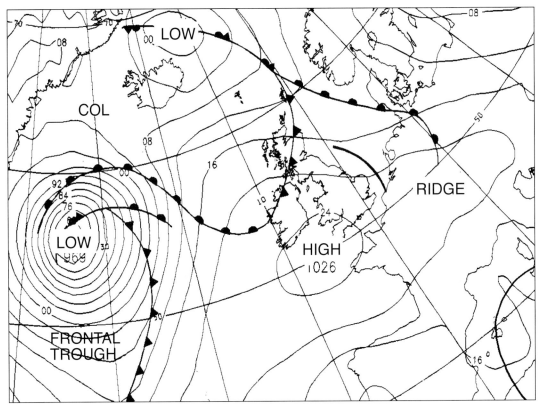

Fig 20.13 *Weatherfax forecast chart.*

Wind

Winds circulate in a clockwise direction around an area of high pressure in the northern hemisphere and clockwise in the southern hemisphere. Winds are lighter and more variable towards the centre of the system. A depression moving towards an anti-cyclone can create a temporary situation with a high pressure gradient and strong winds.

Weather

High pressure systems are associated in summer with settled weather, sunny and warm, clear skies or with little cloud. On the outer part of the system it can be cloudy with perhaps rain. In winter it may be very cold with frost. Radiation fog or mist can occur or there may be complete cloud cover. Sea and land breezes are more noticeable in such a system. In settled weather in summer haze (dust particles) can reduce visibility.

Ridge of high pressure

A ridge of high pressure is a wedge shaped portion of a high pressure system between two low pressure systems. It generally brings fine weather and light winds, Fig 20.13.

Col

A col is a region of intermediate pressure and variable winds between two areas of high pressure and two areas of low pressure. Mist, fog or thunderstorms may occur in a col.

MOTORMASTER

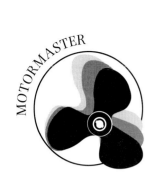

CHAPTER TWENTY ONE

FORECASTING

SOURCES OF WEATHER DATA

Information about weather is obtained from a number of sources, such as a satellite observation station, a land or sea station, or a radiosonde balloon which samples the upper atmosphere. The information is analysed at a national centre, such as the Meteorological Office at Bracknell in England. After analysis the received information is used to produce weather maps in newspapers or on television and radio weather reports and forecasts including the shipping forecast.

A weather map or synoptic chart is a plan showing the relative position of weather systems for the area concerned, together with any associated fronts and other relevant features.

SHIPPING FORECAST

The shipping forecast for waters around the British Isles is broadcast by the British Broadcasting Corporation on Radio 4 (long wave) at 0048, 0555, 1355 and 1750. The wavelength of Radio 4 is 1515 metres which is equivalent to a frequency of 198 kilohertz (198 kHz). Forecasts for other countries are available, details of which can be found in nautical almanacs.

The data from which the shipping forecast is compiled takes quite a while to collect and collate, even with the most up-to-date computers. A shipping forecast broadcast at 1750, although issued by the Meteorological Office at 1700, would be based on an analysis made at 1200. This means that, upon issue, it is already 5 hours out of date and nearly 6 hours out of date when broadcast. This does not mean that the forecast will be incorrect, but there may be some local discrepancies. During unsettled weather, it is sensible to listen for gale warnings broadcast on Radio 4 in the period between shipping forecasts.

Forecasts for inshore waters

The shipping forecast does not take into account local conditions such as land and sea breezes, land configurations or other phenomena, so you will not always experience exactly the weather predicted. Sea area forecasts are also for the centre of the sea area concerned.

After the 0048 shipping forecast there is a forecast for inshore waters which covers waters within 12 miles of the coast around the British Isles. A shorter version of the inshore waters forecast is broadcast on BBC Radio 4 daily at 0550. After the shipping forecast at 0555 and 1750 there are land area forecasts which can give useful additional information mostly concerning sunshine and rain.

Contents of shipping forecast

It is important both to understand the terminology used in various weather forecasts and to be able to make a safe prognosis for a proposed passage. It is usually sufficient to be aware of the position and movement of pressure systems and to make a note of the present and forecast weather in the sea

Fig 21.1 *Shipping forecast map.*

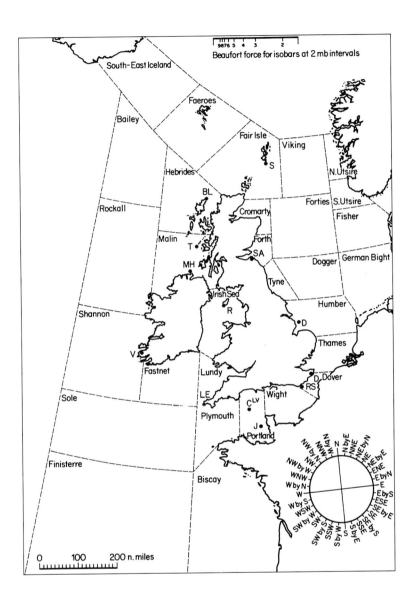

area concerned. During periods of un-settled weather, as conditions can change unexpectedly, it is wise to monitor contin-uously the sources of weather informa-tion supplemented by direct observations.

1 After the initial announcement '*Here is the shipping forecast issued at 1700*', warnings of any gales expected are announced:
'*There are warnings of gales in: Viking,*

North Utsire, South Utsire,...

2 Next comes the general synopsis. This example is valid for 24 hours from 1200 8 March to 1200 9 March. It gives the position of the centre of pres-sure systems with their speed and direction of movement:

'*Here is the general synopsis for 1200: Low 980 North Hebrides moving steadily northeast and filling...*'

TERMS USED IN THE SHIPPING FORECAST

Gale warning

Imminent	=	within 6 hours
Soon	=	between 6 and 12 hours
Later	=	between 12 and 24 hours

Movement of systems

Slowly	=	less than 15 knots
Steadily	=	15 to 25 knots
Rather quickly	=	25 to 35 knots
Rapidly	=	35 to 45 knots
Very rapidly	=	more than 45 knots

Pressure changes

Slowly	=	Change 0.1 to 1.5 mb within 3 hours
Quickly	=	3.5-6 mb within 3 hours
Very rapidly	=	Change of more than 6 mb within 3 hours

Visibility

Very good	=	more than 30 miles
Good	=	5 to 30 miles
Moderate	=	2 to 5 miles
Poor	=	from 1000 m to 2 miles
Mist or haze	=	between 1000 and 2000 m (1100 to 2200 yds)
Fog	=	less than 1000 m (1100 yds)
Thick fog	=	less than 366 m (400 yds)

3 The sea area forecasts are now read out. These are for the 24 hour period from 1700 8 March to 1700 9 March. They cover wind direction and force, weather and visibility:

'*Here are the sea area forecasts: Viking, North Utsire, South Utsire, Forties.*

Southerly 5 becoming northwesterly 7 to 8. Rain then heavy showers. Moderate to poor becoming good...'

4 Lastly reports from coastal stations are given. These are reports of the actual weather at the station at 1600, giving wind direction and force, weather, visibility, pressure and pressure tendency:

'*Here are the reports from coastal stations for 1600: Tiree, west by north 7, fair, 11 miles, 1000, rising rapidly...*'

The information broadcast in the shipping forecast can be tape recorded for plotting later or it can be taken down on a prepared form, but due to the speed with which it is read it is necessary to use some form of shorthand such as the Beaufort notation shown at the end of this chapter.

RADIO AIDS TO WEATHER FORECASTING

Navtex

NAVTEX is an international telex service broadcast on 518kHz. You will need a receiver that can operate on this frequency, together with a small printer. NAVTEX can provide navigational warnings, weather forecasts, gale warnings and search and rescue information.

Fig 21.2 shows a NAVTEX Shipping Forecast timed at 0818 on 18 April. The general synopsis at midnight reports a low 985 southeast Iceland moving rather quickly east.

Weatherfax

Weatherfax is a service which provides, via a radio receiver modem and printer, weather information such as: surface analysis, surface weather, forecasts for 24, 48 and

MOTORMASTER

72 hours ahead, gale warnings in force, surface wind and a sea and swell prognoses.

Fig 21.3 shows surface winds at 0600 on 18 April; Fig 21.4 shows surface weather at 0600 on 18 April.

Use of Weatherfax

NAVTEX and Weatherfax outputs, such as those shown above, can be used when planning a passage.

What might be the constraints on a passage from Lymington to Poole and back during the afternoon of 18 April?

The forecast from Radio Niton for sea area Wight at 0700 on 18 April indicates: wind, westerly 4 or 5; weather, mainly fair; visibility, moderate with fog patches. From Fig 21.3 the surface wind forecast at 0600 on 18 April indicates: westerly 5 (initially slightly north of west).

From Fig 21.2 the general synopsis at midnight (17 April) is: Low 985 Southeast Iceland, moving rather quickly east (25 to 35 knots) expected Sweden 976 by midnight tonight (18 April). High West Finisterre 1041 expected East Finisterre 1034 by same time.

By 1200 on 18 April, the low has moved as forecast at about 30 knots and is occluding. The high is declining with little movement. The wind is likely to remain westerly 4 to 5 for the next 12 hours.

The wave height will depend on the strength and direction of the tidal stream. A strong tidal stream against the wind and over shoal waters will result in rough seas, especially to the west of the Needles lighthouse. The visibility will be moderate but look out for fog patches.

An afternoon passage from Lymington to Poole and back is quite feasible, though expect lively seas off the Needles. There is always the option to return to Lymington if the sea is too rough.

```
NITON RADIO
SHIPPING FORECAST

0818 ON SATURDAY 18 APRIL

THE GENERAL SYNOPSIS AT MIDNIGHT
LOW 985 SOUTHEAST ICELAND MOVING
RATHER QUICKLY EAST EXPECTED
SWEDEN 976 BY MIDNIGHT TONIGHT. HIGH
WEST FINISTERRE 1041 EXPECTED
EAST FINISTERRE 1034 BY SAME TIME.

THE AREA FORECASTS FOR THE NEXT 24
HOURS
ISSUED BY THE
METEOROLOGICAL OFFICE AT 180700 GMT

THAMES DOVER WIGHT PORTLAND
PLYMOUTH BISCAY
WESTERLY 4 OR 5. MAINLY FAIR. MODERATE
WITH FOG PATCHES

SOUTH FINISTERRE
NORTHEASTERLY 4 OR 5 VEERING EASTERLY
4. FAIR. GOOD

NORTH FINISTERRE SOLE
WESTERLY 4 OR 5, BACKING SOUTHERLY 4
OR 5 IN WEST LATER. FAIR.
MODERATE WITH FOG PATCHES

LUNDY FASTNET IRISH SEA SHANNON
WEST OR SOUTHWEST 4 OR 5. FAIR.
MODERATE WITH FOG PATCHES

ROCKALL MALIN
SOUTHWESTERLY 5 TO 7, OCCASIONALLY
GALE 8 IN NORTH ROCKALL AT FIRST,
BECOMING VARIABLE 4 IN NORTH. RAIN AT
TIMES. MODERATE WITH FOG PATCHES,
BECOMING GOOD IN NORTH
```

Fig 21.2 *NAVTEX shipping forecast.*

MOTORMASTER

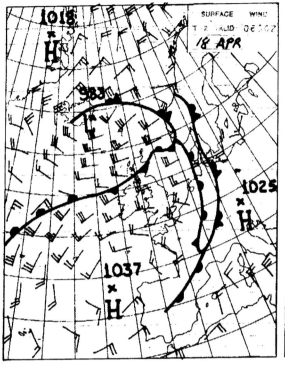

Fig 21.3 *Surface winds (extract from original fax).*

Fig 21.4 *Surface weather (extract from original fax).*

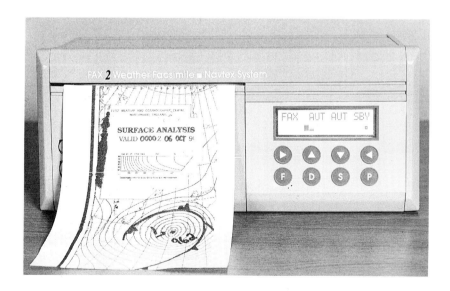

Weather facsimile. Navtex system.

MetFAX Marine

MetFAX Marine is a dial-up fax forecast and weather service provided by the Met. Office. Anyone with access to a fax machine can request Met. Office information and forecasts immediately and automatically.

The fax machine is set to the POLL RECEIVE mode, without documents in the feeder, before dialling one of the product numbers. For fax machines which have a handset, dial the product number and press the START button when instructed to do so.

MetFAX Marine is a premium rate telephone service. Details of the product numbers and costs can be obtained by dialling 0336-400-401.

Figs 21.5 to 21.8 show a sequence of Surface Analysis and Surface Forecast charts for the period 1200 GMT Monday 18 Jan to 1200 GMT Thursday 21 Jan. Fig 21.9 shows the forecast for the English Channel over the same period.

If you were thinking of crossing the English Channel from the Isle of Wight to the Channel Islands, examination of the charts would give you the following information:

1 Monday 18 Jan (Fig 21.5). There is a southwesterly airstream of about 20 knots (force 5) along the English Channel. (The wind speed can be deduced from the geostrophic wind scale. However a simple rule-of-thumb is that, if the distance between isobars spaced at 4 mb intervals is the same as the distance from Land's End to North Foreland, ie the length of the south coast of England, the wind speed will be 10 knots. Halving the distance between the isobars doubles the wind speed.) To the west of Ireland there is a low (1006 mb) approaching with an associated occluded front. From Fig 21.6 (24 hours later), this low is 996 mb just west of Denmark so the front will probably pass over around midnight. Note that, by following the isobars westward, the air mass is predominantly from the southwest so the weather should be mild.

2 Tuesday 19 Jan (Fig 21.6). The southwesterly airstream continues but the approaching frontal system to the west of Ireland heralds stronger winds and persistent rain by late evening.

3 Wednesday 20 Jan (Fig 21.7). The airstream is now westerly and probably up to gale force on the passage of the fronts. The wind could moderate for a while after midnight with clearing skies.

4 Thursday 21 Jan (Fig 21.8). Though the wind is about 25 knots (force 6) from the west or southwest and the weather is clear, there is another frontal system approaching which will bring rain followed by drizzle and poor visibility. The wind could back to southwest and increase to 30 knots (force 7) early on Friday morning.

Fig 21.9 is the associated forecast which correlates with the deductions above. Note that the sea state becomes progressively rougher with the persistent strong winds from the west.

Any passage across the English Channel would be uncomfortable, which is not surprising in January. There is a ridge of high pressure over France which suggests that a passage across the Bay of Biscay during the same period could be quite feasible and possibly even a little windless towards the south.

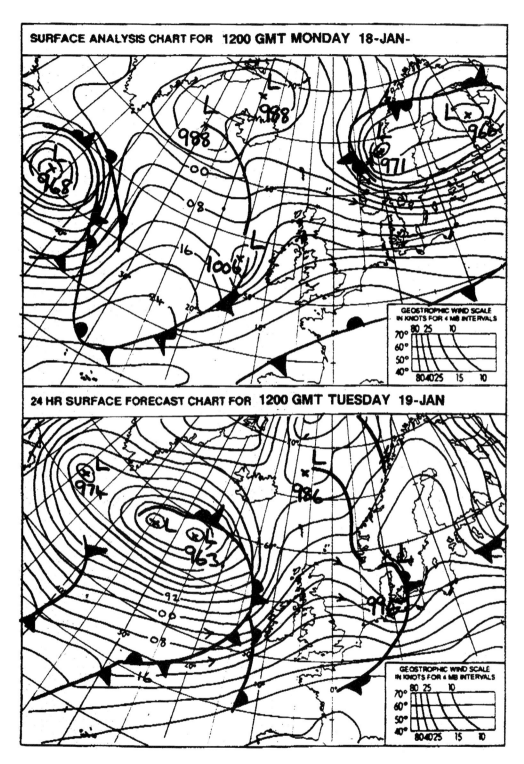

Fig 21.5 and 21.6 *Met FAX surface analysis charts (extracts from original fax).*

MOTORMASTER

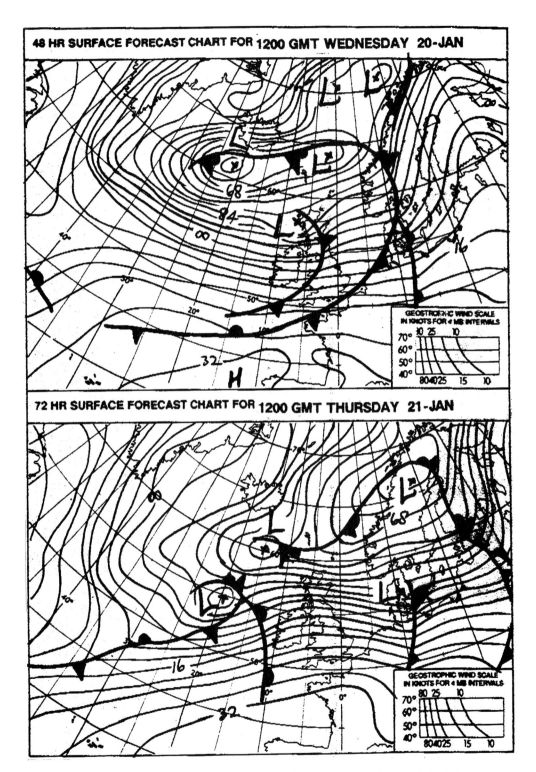

Fig 21.7 and 21.8 *METFAX surface analysis charts (extracts from original fax).*

Fig 21.9 *This detailed and informative text accompanies the synoptic charts seen on page 161-62. Notice how the sea state becomes progressively rougher due to the strong winds from the west.*

FORECAST FOR THE AREA LYME REGIS TO SELSEY BILL
AND 12 MILES OFFSHORE, ISSUED BY THE MET OFFICE,
SOUTHAMPTON WEATHER CENTRE AT 7PM ON MONDAY 18TH JANUARY
FOR THE PERIOD ENDING AT 7AM ON WEDNESDAY

GENERAL SITUATION

DESPITE AN AREA OF HIGH PRESSURE ON THE NEAR CONTINENT, CENTRED
OVER GERMANY, LOW PRESSURE WILL PASS CLOSE TO NORTHERN IRELAND
TONIGHT, PUSHING AN ATLANTIC FRONT EASTWARDS OVERNIGHT, AND
MAINTAINING THE WINDY, UNSETTLED SPELL OF WEATHER.

FORECAST UNTIL 7PM ON TUESDAY

WIND : SOUTH OR SOUTHWESTERLY FORCE 5, INCREASING FORCE 6 THIS
EVENING, BUT REACHING FORCE 7 ROUND EXPOSED HEADLANDS. VEERING
WESTERLY AND REDUCING FORCE 4 BY THE EARLY HOURS, BUT BACKING
SOUTHWESTERLY BY MIDDAY AND INCREASING FORCE 5 OR 6 BY THE EVENING.

WEATHER : CLOUD AND RAIN SOON SPREADING EAST, BUT CLEARING BY THE
EARLY HOURS TO CLEAR OR SUNNY SPELLS ON TUESDAY MORNING. CLOUD
INCREASING DURING THE AFTERNOON, WITH SOME LIGHT RAIN BY EVENING.

VISIBILITY : MODERATE AT FIRST AND LATER, BUT MAINLY GOOD.

SEA STATE : MODERATE OR ROUGH INCREASING ROUGH OR VERY ROUGH BY THE
EARLY HOURS. MAINLY ROUGH ON TUESDAY.

SURF : 4 TO 6 FEET ON TUESDAY, HIGHEST IN LYME BAY.

MAXIMUM AIR TEMPERATURE : 9 DEGREES CELSIUS

SEA TEMPERATURE : 10 DEGREES CELSIUS

FORECAST FROM 7PM ON TUESDAY UNTIL 7AM WEDNESDAY

WIND : SOUTHWESTERLY FORCE 6 INCREASING FORCE 7 TO GALE FORCE 8
WITH GUSTS TO 50 KNOTS BY MIDNIGHT.

WEATHER : CLOUDY WITH RAIN, HEAVY AT TIMES.

VISIBILITY : MODERATE, PERHAPS POOR AFTER MIDNIGHT WEST OF POOLE
BAY.

SEA STATE : ROUGH INCREASING VERY ROUGH AFTER MIDNIGHT.

THIS IS THE 3 TO 5 DAY FORECAST FOR THE ENGLISH CHANNEL FOR THE
AREA BETWEEN LANDS END AND ROSCOFF, AND NORTH FORELAND AND
DUNKERQUE, ISSUED BY THE MET OFFICE, SOUTHAMPTON WEATHER CENTRE
AT 4AM ON MONDAY 18TH JANUARY
THIS FORECAST IS FROM WEDNESDAY UNTIL FRIDAY

GENERAL SITUATION

THE VERY MOBILE AND UNSETTLED PATTERN WILL PERSIST THROUGHOUT THE FORECAST PERIOD. DEEP ATLANTIC DEPRESSIONS WILL KEEP PRESSURE LOW TO THE NORTH OF SCOTLAND AS MAJOR CENTRES PASS NORTHEASTWARDS THROUGH THE ICELAND-FAROES GAP. ASSOCIATED WEATHER FRONTS WILL SWEEP ACROSS THE BRITISH ISLES DURING THE PERIOD BRINGING BELTS OF RAIN AND STRONG OR GALE FORCE WINDS TO CHANNEL WATERS FROM TIME TO TIME.

FORECAST FOR WEDNESDAY

WIND : SOUTH TO SOUTHWESTERLY FORCE 4 OR 5, INCREASING TO FORCE 6 OR 7 DURING THE MORNING EARLY, AND PERHAPS TO GALE FORCE 8 FOR A TIME IMMEDIATELY AHEAD OF A COLD FRONT MOVING EAST TO CLEAR THE CHANNEL BY EARLY AFTERNOON. WINDS WILL VEER SOUTHWESTERLY BEHIND THIS COLD FRONT AND WILL DECREASE FORCE 6 AT FIRST BUT FORCE 5 BY DUSK.

WEATHER : CLOUDY CONDITIONS WITH OUTBREAKS OF DRIZZLE AT FIRST, BUT A BELT OF MORE PERSISTENT RAIN REACHING LANDS END TO ROSCOFF SOON AFTER DAWN WILL SPREAD EAST THROUGH ALL WATERS DURING THE MORNING. CLEARER CONDITIONS, BUT WITH A FEW SHOWERS, FOLLOWING ON, AND REACHING THE STRAIT OF DOVER BY EARLY AFTERNOON.

VISIBILITY : MODERATE TO POOR, IN DRIZZLE AND RAIN, BECOMING GOOD IN THE CLEARER WEATHER FOLLOWING.

SEA STATE : MODERATE INCREASING ROUGH OR VERY ROUGH DURING THE MORNING. SUBSIDING SLOWLY IN THE CLEARER WEATHER BUT STILL MODERATE TO ROUGH.

FORECAST FOR THURSDAY

WIND : SOUTHWESTERLY FORCE 5 OR 6, AND INCREASING FORCE 7 GENERALLY, BUT GALE FORCE 8 IN PLACES DURING THE AFTERNOON. BACKING SOUTH OR SOUTHWEST DURING THE EVENING.

WEATHER : SCATTERED SHOWERS AT FIRST. A SPELL OF MAINLY LIGHT RAIN SPREADING EAST DURING THE AFTERNOON AND EVENING, WITH PATCHY DRIZZLE SUBSEQUENTLY.

VISIBILITY : GOOD, BECOMING MODERATE TO POOR DURING THE AFTERNOON, WITH PATCHY SEA FOG LIKELY FROM EVENING, EAST OF ISLE OF WIGHT.

SEA STATE :   ROUGH INCREASING VERY ROUGH DURING THE MORNING.

FORECAST FOR FRIDAY

WIND : SOUTH TO SOUTHWESTERLY FORCE 7 TO GALE FORCE 8, AND PERHAPS SEVERE GALE FORCE 9 IN OPEN WATERS AT TIMES.

WEATHER : CLOUDY WITH OCCASIONAL DRIZZLE.

VISIBILITY : MODERATE TO POOR, BUT VERY POOR IN ODD PATCHES OF SEA FOG

SEA STATE : VERY ROUGH TO HIGH.

Fig 21.9 *Continued.*

MOTORMASTER

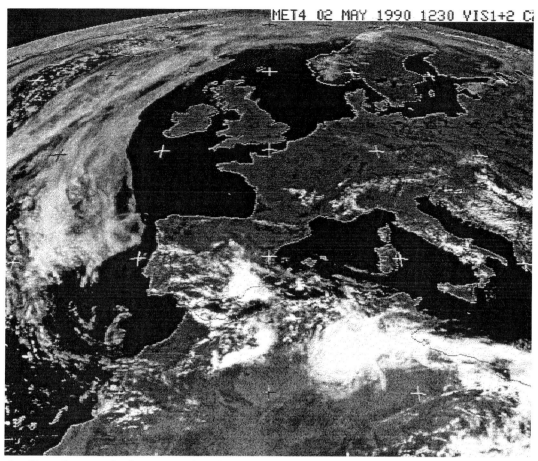

MET4 02 MAY 1990 1230 VIS1+2 C

Satellite photograph showing a clear band of high pressure over Europe and a front moving across from the west.

Weather Satellites

Weather satellites relay cloud pictures. The photo above shows a typical satellite picture, showing cloud over the Atlantic and North Africa with clear skies over Europe. The weather satellites are in geo-stationary orbit 23,000 miles above the Equator. One of these satellites METEO-STAT, provides satellite pictures of Europe, Africa and the Middle East.

The following types of image are available via METEO-STAT:

• Images (infra red) of the whole of Europe every 30 minutes.

• Visible light close-ups of Europe every hour during daylight hours.

• Pictures of the Atlantic, Middle East and Africa at less frequent intervals.

• Infra red pictures of North, Central and South America retransmitted from the American GOES weather satellite.

• Whole earth pictures 16 times a day. Normally weather satellite information is received using a dish antenna with a receiver unit and displayed on an IBM compatible personal computer using a VGA monitor.

MOTORMASTER

BEAUFORT WIND SCALE

Force	Description	Limit of mean wind speed (kts)	Appearance	Approx wave height (m)
0	Calm	less than 1	Sea like a mirror.	0
1	Light airs	1 to 3	Ripples like scales.	less than 0.1
2	Light breeze	4 to 6	Small wavelets. Crests have a glassy appearance but do not break	0.1 to 0.3
3	Gentle breeze	7 to 10	Large wavelets. A few white horses.	0.3 to 0.9
4	Moderate breeze	11 to 16	Small waves becoming longer. Frequent white horses.	0.9 to 1.5
5	Fresh breeze	17 to 21	Moderate waves. Many white horses.	1.5 to 2.5
6	Strong breeze	22 to 27	Large waves. White foam crests. Some spray.	2.5 to 4
7	Near gale	28 to 33	Sea heaps up. Waves break. Streaks of foam.	4 to 6
8	Gale	34 to 40	Moderately high waves of greater length. Crests breaking into spindrift. Extensive streaks of foam.	6 to 8
9	Severe gale	41 to 47	High waves. Dense streaks of foam. Crests begin to topple. Spray affects visibility.	8 to 10
10	Storm	48 to 55	Very high waves with overhanging crests. Dense white streaks of foam. Tumbling sea. Visibility affected.	10 to 12
11	Violent storm	56 to 63	Extremely high waves. Sea completely covered with patches of foam. Edges of wave crests blown into froth. Visibility affected.	12 to 14
12	Hurricane	64 to 71	Air filled with foam and spray. Sea completely white with driving spray. Visibility very seriously affected.	14 to 16

OTHER SOURCES OF WEATHER INFORMATION

Coast Radio Stations

These are maintained by British Telecom International as a radio telephone service. They broadcast at set times the portion of the last shipping forecast for their own area, gale warnings and the general synopsis, including any changes which may have occurred since the main shipping forecast. These are broadcast on the VHF maritime frequency band. Details of times and channels are found in Admiralty Lists of Radio Signals and in nautical almanacs.

Local Radio Stations

Both BBC and independent local radio stations often repeat a portion of the shipping forecast covering their own area.

Land Weather Forecasts

Radio forecasts for the weather on land are useful, although they concentrate on rain and sunshine rather than wind and visibility., They often give the general trend for a day or two ahead and can provide background information to complement the shipping forecast.

Telephone Recorded Forecasts

Marinecall forecasts give information provided by the Meteorological Office for coastal areas around the British Isles for distances up to 12 nautical miles off the coastline. They are updated two or three

---

USEFUL EXTRACTS
FROM THE BEAUFORT NOTATION

d	drizzle	r	rain
f	fog	rs	sleet
h	hail	s	snow
l	lightning	t	thunder
m	mist	tl	thunderstorms
q	squalls	z	haze

Capital letters are used to indicate 'intense'.

Double letters are used to indicate 'continuous'.

The prefix 'i' indicates 'intermittent'.

The prefix 'p' indicates 'passing' showers.

The suffix [o] indicates 'slight'.

The solidus '/' indicates a time interval.

MOTORMASTER

times daily. The information includes sea state and relevant high water times.

Weathercall forecasts give a similar service but cover land areas. A time check is included in both services.

TV and Newspapers

These give weather charts and analysis, with a prognosis for the following day and sometimes satellite pictures. This is useful background information if studied a day or two before a proposed passage.

Local Weather Centres

Forecasts from local Weather Centres can be obtained by radio telephone when at sea or by telephone or personal visit when ashore. Weekend packs are available for mariners at some Weather Centres, with forecast charts for 3 days ahead.

Local Information

It is valuable to talk to local water users such as fishermen, marina berthing masters, harbour masters and yacht clubs to obtain local information.

Coastguard

The United Kingdom Coastguard broadcasts weather forecasts from information supplied by the Meteorological Office at regular intervals on VHF radio channel 67.

Small Craft Warnings

These are issued by the Meteorological Office between April and October when winds of force 6 or more are expected up to 5 miles from shore during the next 12 hours. They are broadcast by the BBC and independent radio stations, usually after the first programme break after reception and repeated following the next news bulletin.

Gale Warnings

Gale warnings for all home waters are broadcast on BBC Radio 4, 198kHz, when winds of force 8 or more are expected. They are issued as soon as possible after receipt and repeated after the next news bulletin. Coast Radio Stations also broadcast gale warnings.

QUESTIONS

Use the extracts provided in this chapter.

21.1 A navigator is about to plan a passage. Where can he obtain:
a) Details of the present and forecast weather including wind strength and direction, visibility and sea state.
b) Details of the position and movement of weather systems likely to affect the passage together with details of any gale warnings.

21.2 The morning shipping forecast at 0555 was missed. Where can details of gale warnings, general synopsis, sea area forecast and reports from coastal stations for a passage from Yarmouth (Isle of Wight) to Swanage be obtained?

21.3 The wind has been blowing southwest 6 to 7 for the past two days but has now veered to northwest 5. A 19 m shallow draught motorboat with a cruising speed of 8 knots proposes to leave Poole Harbour on the ebb tide at spring tides and round Anvil Point on passage westwards, Fig 21.10. Is it wise to make the proposed passage or should the start be postponed?

21.4 What do the following terms mean?
a) **Poor** visibility.
b) A depression moving **rapidly**.
c) A **near gale**.
d) A **moderate** breeze.
e) **Later**.

21.5 The following is an extract from a shipping forecast:

General synopsis. Low Viking moving steadily northeast.

Sea area forecast. Wight: southwest 5 becoming northwest 6 to 8 decreasing 5 later; poor becoming good.

Reports from coastal stations. Dover: southwest 5, rain, 2 miles, 1012, steady. Channel Light Vessel: northwest 8, showers, 12 miles, 1012, rising rapidly.

a) What feature will shortly pass over sea area Wight?
b) With reference to the following, describe the changes which will occur in sea area Wight over the next 24 hours: wind strength and direction; barometric pressure; visibility; precipitation; cloud; temperature.
c) You are proposing a passage from Cherbourg to Southampton. When do you think you should plan to depart?

21.6 Here is an extract from the Shipping Forecast broadcast at 0555:

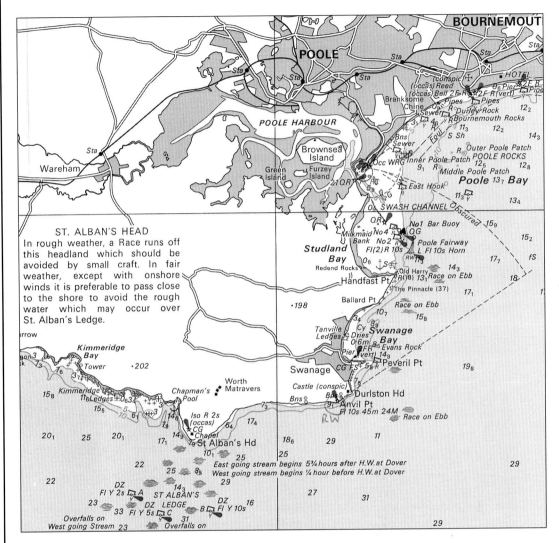

Fig 21.10.

Wind southwest 4 to 6 increasing 7 becoming northwest 7 to 8 later; rain; visibility poor becoming good.

Your destination is the island shown in Fig 21.11 which is in the sea area concerned.

List the three anchorages shown in order of preference:
a) To stop for lunch.
b) To stay overnight.
Give your reasons.

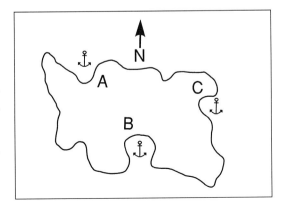

Fig 21.11.

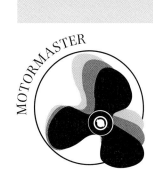

CHAPTER TWENTY TWO

SAFETY AT SEA

There are always risks to water users as with any other sporting activity. However to minimise these risks it is important to have on board the correct safety equipment and to know when and how to use it. The skipper must always be aware of the capabilities both of the boat and of the crew and must plan the proposed passage accordingly, paying due attention to expected weather.

Boats above 13.7 m (45 ft) in length are subject to regulations which require them to carry certain items of safety equipment. Merchant Shipping Regulations are available from Her Majesty's Stationery Office.

PERSONAL SAFETY EQUIPMENT

- Warm clothing including hat, gloves, a change of clothing, oilskins and waterproof non-slip footwear.

- A lifejacket with light for each person on board to BS3595 specification, to be worn should there be a danger of the boat sinking, and when in the tender (dinghy). Every year a number of drownings occur between the boat and the shore.

- Personal survival beacon.

- A safety harness to BS4474 specification is not as essential on a motorboat as for a sailing boat where crew members are constantly on the foredeck often in rough weather. Most motor craft have safety rails and grab rails. However, it is

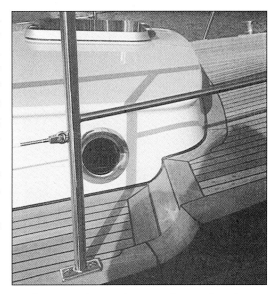

Make sure that pulpits and guard rails are securely fixed to the deck.

recommended that at least two safety harnesses be kept ready for use should it be necessary for crew to be on the foredeck at night or in rough weather, or if using an outside steering position. Strong attachments for harnesses should be placed in such a position as to prevent a person from falling into the water, as at even a speed of 8 knots, anyone going over the side whilst attached to the boat could break their back.

- A sharp knife to cut any ropes which may be a hazard.

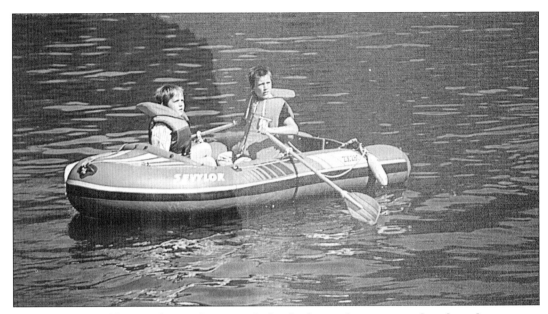

Your children will love to play in the cruiser's dinghy but make very sure that they always wear life jackets.

CHECKLIST OF GENERAL SAFETY EQUIPMENT

- A liferaft of an approved type (USCG or SOLAS) with a capacity to carry all persons on board. This should be readily accessible and easy to launch. It should be tested every year by a qualified test centre.

  Most cases of liferaft launchings are not due to rough weather, but collision and fire. It is more economical to rent a liferaft unless it is needed for the whole year as this way there are no service charges.

- At least two lifebuoys, one with a self igniting light and drogue and one with 30 m of floating line. A deck quoit with floating line attached is also useful as a heaving line when dealing with a man overboard situation. A U shaped lifebelt is best as it will fit under the arms.

- A dan buoy with a self igniting light. A lifebuoy with drogue can be attached to this.

- A boarding ladder. Such ladders are usually fitted to the stern of the boat which is a convenient place for a swimming platform or for boarding the tender but not a good place to recover a man from the water as the stern of the boat may be moving up and down considerably in rough weather, and it is near the propellers. It is a good idea, therefore, to carry an additional ladder to lower over the side in an emergency. This can be a rope ladder or scrambling net suitably weighted down.

- Two buckets with strong handles and lanyards for use as bailers or for fire fighting.

- At least two multi-purpose fire extinguishers of a suitable capacity with a minimum rating of 5A/34B to BS5423.

Additionally, for high powered engines, an automatic or semi-automatic fire fighting system fitted in the engine compartment or engine room.

- A fire blanket BS6575.

- Navigation lights and a searchlight.

- At least two anchors of sufficient size with sufficient chain and warp for all expected depths and conditions.

- A waterproof torch.

- A piece of canvas with the boat's name to be displayed in an emergency.

- A method of securing all heavy gear, including batteries, liable to do damage by coming loose in heavy weather.

- A radio suitable for receiving the shipping forecast.

- Marine band radio: VHF or MF. A hand-held VHF radio.

- Radar reflector, preferably permanently fixed; or radar target enhancer.

- Radar.

- Electronic position fixing system such as Decca, GPS.

- Efficient steering compass and a hand-bearing compass.

- Reliable clock and watch; stop-watch.

- Distance log.

- Echo sounder.

- Barometer.

- Lead line.

- Charts and relevant nautical publications corrected to date.

- Plotting instruments.

- Tool kit including engine tools and bolt croppers.

- Engine spares.

- Separate batteries for engine starting.

- Tow rope.

- Tender (dinghy)

- Spare fuel.

- Gas warning system.

- Fixed and portable bilge pump neither of which rely on electrical power.

- A horn for sound signalling.

- Flares.

- First aid kit.

- Mooring warps and fenders.

- Emergency water supply isolated from the main fresh water tanks.

- Emergency position indicating radio beacon (EPIRB).

Stowage

All equipment should have its own place on the boat and be kept in that place so that it can be found at any time without a lengthy search. This is particularly important when it is dark or in rough weather. All safety equipment such as liferaft, life jackets, safety harnesses, flares and first aid kits should be readily accessible. Fire extinguishers should be near exits and the fire blanket near but not over the cooker. A stowage list of equipment should be prominently displayed, but people unfamiliar with the boat should be shown where everything is soon after they come on board.

MOTORMASTER

Maintenance

Regular inspection and maintenance of all equipment is essential. Any out-of-date items should be replaced or serviced immediately. The engine should be serviced regularly. Preferably a sea-going motorboat should have two independent engines each with its own electrical system and separate battery.

Even an efficiently working engine is no use if there is a fouled propeller. It is a good idea to keep diving equipment on board and a diver's knife ready to deal with this possibility.

LIFERAFTS

Liferafts should be of an approved type and satisfy the conditions laid down by such authorities as the United States Coast Guard (USCG), or Safety of Life At Sea (SOLAS) which is a working committee of the International Maritime Organisation (IMO).

Everyone on board should know where the liferaft is stowed, how to launch it and how to board it. Some interesting features and equipment are listed on page 175.

Preparation for Launch

1 Do not launch the liferaft until it is needed as it could turn over or become damaged if towed behind. Send a MAYDAY distress call on the VHF radio before launching (see page 118).

2 Secure the painter (line) of the liferaft to a strong point on the boat.

3 Unlash the raft and remove from its stowage.

4 Launch overboard and stand clear of the painter.

5 When the raft is in the water, take in the slack on the painter and tug sharply to inflate.

6 If possible put on or collect extra warm clothing.

7 Put on lifejackets.

8 Collect the portable VHF radio and the EPIRB if these are on board. Activate the EPIRB after acknowledgement of MAYDAY distress call.

Boarding

• Do not leave the boat for the liferaft until it is absolutely necessary to do so, as it provides protection and is a bigger target for the rescue authorities to spot.

• Get into the raft dry, if possible. Do not jump in. If it is necessary to enter the water, do this in front of the raft and spend as little time as possible in the water. Conserve energy.

• Get a strong person in first to help the others.

After Boarding

• When everyone has left the boat, cut the painter and paddle away from the boat. If there are any survivors still in the water, paddle towards them; throw a heaving line and pull them in. Stream the drogue (sea anchor).

• Activate the EPIRB.

• Check for leaks and fit leak stoppers if required. If necessary top up the buoyancy chambers with the pump.

• Open the survival pack. Take out first aid kit, flares and anti-seasickness tablets. Treat any injuries, and issue anti seasickness tablets.

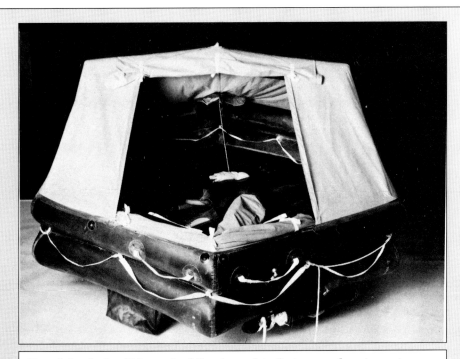

Your liferaft should have the following safety features and equipment: a canopy which is automatically erected and has a vent and external light; upper and lower independent buoyancy chambers inflated by a CO_2 cylinder; pockets underneath to hold water for stabilization; grab handles and a lifeline; bailer, paddles, pump and hose; and emergency grab bag including a first aid kit, repair kit, fishing kit, space blanket, survival rations; can opener, a container of drinking water with cup; knife, whistle; flares; personal EPIRB; drogue or sea anchor; torch. Photo: Beaufort Air-Sea Equipment Ltd.

- Post a look-out with flares at hand and work out a watch system.
- Ration water and do not issue any for 24 hours unless anyone is injured and losing blood. Do not drink sea water or urine. It is not a good idea to eat protein food if there is a shortage of water as it needs plenty of water to digest it.
- If a rescue vessel or helicopter is approaching, pin-point your position with a red handflare or day smoke.
- Anyone being sick should use the bag provided and not lean out of the raft.

MOTORMASTER

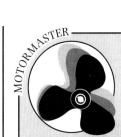

FIRE EXTINGUISHERS

A fire needs three elements for it to take hold and spread:

- Fuel
- Oxygen
- Heat

The most efficient way to deal with a fire is to starve it of one or all of these three elements. Fire extinguishers are designed to do just that. Different classes of extinguisher are more efficient on certain types of fire. Those manufactured to BS5423 are coded with a letter to denote the class of fire for which they are most suitable and a number to indicate their capacity.

Class A This is for use with carbonaceous material such as paper, textiles, wood. Extinguishers containing water, foam or powder are all suitable. Water can of course be poured on from a bucket.

Be aware that the fire may appear to be out but can smoulder and restart later. If water is used, the material and the surrounding area must be thoroughly soaked. Water is a good medium for this type of a fire but, due to its surface tension, it does not necessarily penetrate the material, so the addition of a simple detergent helps.

Class B This is for use with flammable liquids such as petrol, cooking oil, paraffin and paint materials. Extinguishers containing powder, CO_2 gas or foam are suitable. Do not use water as it spreads the fire.

Class C This is for flammable gases such as propane or butane. Extinguishers containing powder or CO_2 gas are suitable but not water or foam.

Water
This contains a gas cartridge and water is sprayed out under pressure. Aim at the base of the fire and thoroughly soak the surrounding area. The water has a cooling effect on the fire. It is fairly effective on wood, textiles and paper but should *not* be used on electrical fires.

Spray Foam
This is filled with aqueous film-forming foam (AFFF) and contains a gas cartridge. Foam is sprayed out under pressure. It smothers the flame and prevents re-ignition of flammable vapours by sealing the surface. This is effective on engine room fires but not on electrical fires.

Dry Powder
This contains powder under pressure. It retards the combustion process and melts to form a seal which prevents flammable vapours rising from the surface. This is possibly the best, cheapest all-round extinguisher for use on a boat as you can tackle most kinds of fire.

Carbon Dioxide Gas (CO$_2$)

This is a pressurised cylinder of CO$_2$ gas. It works by depriving flames of oxygen and is effective on flammable liquids. It should be directed at the fire. It is not particularly suitable for boats because large capacity extinguishers are needed which are bulky.

Halon

Halon gas is a very effective extinguishing medium, probably one of the best for electrical fires. Unfortunately it is an ozone depleting gas and has consequently been banned in a number of countries.

Fire Blanket

An efficient way to deal with a cooker fire is to smother it with a fire blanket BS6575, or use a heavy damp piece of material. This will starve the fire of oxygen. The blanket should be placed on the fire away from the person holding it so that the flames are not fanned. It should be left for 10 minutes. A blazing pan should never be thrown overboard as there is a danger of spillage which can cause a more serious fire.

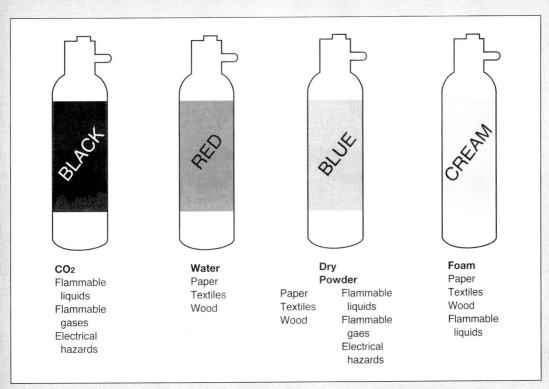

CO$_2$	**Water**	**Dry Powder**		**Foam**
Flammable liquids	Paper		Flammable liquids	Paper
Flammable gases	Textiles	Paper	Flammable gaes	Textiles
Electrical hazards	Wood	Textiles	Electrical hazards	Wood
		Wood		Flammable liquids

A quick reference chart showing the colour code and type of extinguisher needed for each kind of fire. For electrical fires use dry powder or CO$_2$ but not water or foam.

FIRE PREVENTION

Prevention is always better than cure. Simple safety precautions will considerably minimise the risk of fire.

Refuelling

- Stop the engine and turn off the fuel supply.

- Turn off the cooker, lighting equipment and heaters. Extinguish all naked flames and do not smoke.

- Close all openings below deck.

- Monitor the amount of fuel in the tank and see that it does not overflow.

After Refuelling

- See that the fuel cap is tightly secured.

- Check that the fuel has not overflowed.

- Clean up any spills and wash over the side, using detergent if necessary.

- Ventilate the boat before re-starting the engine or using naked flames.

Spare Fuel

- Only fill fuel cans in the open air. Take the same precautions as when filling the fuel tank.

- Only use containers specially designed for carrying fuel.

- Fix containers securely away from engine, exhaust, cooker, heaters or cabin accommodation.

Gas

- See that the cooker, gas cylinder and interconnecting pipes are properly fitted.

- Gas cylinders should be in a compartment which ventilates overboard.

- When the cooker is used, the valve on the cylinder is turned on first and then the knob on the cooker. When finished with, it is turned off from the bottle first and then the cooker to allow any unused gas in the pipe to burn away. Some systems have a fail-safe fitted so that the knob on the cooker has to be held pushed-in for a few seconds after lighting to heat a thermocouple which allows gas to flow through. This means that if the knob is accidentally knocked on or the gas blows out, no gas will escape.

- Always turn off the gas at the cylinder when not in use, particularly overnight.

- Do not leave a lit cooker unattended.

- When changing a cylinder, turn the valve on the cylinder to the *off* position before removing the cylinder. Replace with the full cylinder and turn on. Test for leaks by smearing water and soap around the join between valve and cylinder. If bubbles appear, there is a gas leak.

FIRE

1 If a fire breaks out on the boat alert everyone by shouting '**FIRE**'.

2 Attack the fire with the nearest fire extinguisher aiming at the base of the fire. Turn off gas and fuel supply. Move any fuel containers and gas cylinders to a safe place even if it means disconnecting the gas cylinders. If necessary, for the boat's safety, dispose of these overboard.

3 Get everyone, apart from those fighting the fire, up on deck. The main danger with a fire below is being trapped. For this reason fire extinguishers should be near exits so that an escape route is available if needed.

4 If the fire appears to be getting out of hand, put on life jackets, launch the tender and tow it behind and prepare the liferaft ready for launching. Get ready to alert the rescue services and initiate distress procedures.

5 If things get out of control, do not risk life, abandon the boat and move away from it.

suspected gas leak

Stop the engine.

Extinguish all flames.

Turn off the fuel and gas at source.

Ventilate the boat by opening all doors and portholes.

Do not use the engine, cooker, heater or naked flames until the leak has been stopped and the boat has been ventilated.

eneral

A boat which has not been used for a while should be thoroughly ventilated before use.

Keep bilges and engine compartment clean.

Do not smoke in the berth and take care where cigarette ends, used matches and pipe ash are disposed of.

See that everyone on board knows where the fire appliances are stowed and knows how to use them. By taking the correct action promptly, a major disaster can usually be averted.

Fit a gas detector.

HELICOPTER RESCUE

- A boat in distress may not be easily identified from the air and should, therefore, be clearly marked with her name on a piece of canvas spread across the deck.

- If the helicopter is in the vicinity and the boat thinks she has not been seen, a red flare can be fired or an orange smoke ignited. Do not fire the flare in the direction of the helicopter. If using smoke flares see that smoke does not get into the cockpit of the helicopter.

- Clear the deck or tie down any objects which may be blown about by the strong downrush of air from the rotor blades.

- Do not leave the boat until instructed to do so. If you have to leave the boat, wear lifejackets, and, if you can, get into the liferaft, or the dinghy. These can be attached to the boat using a long line.

- The boat's drift should be minimised by the use of a sea anchor.

- Because of the danger of static electricity, do not touch the winch wire. Don't attempt to attach it to the boat. Instructions will be given by the helicopter and usually one of the helicopter crew is winched down to the boat.

Aircraft looking for vessels in distress or liferafts fly a search pattern during which they may fire a green pyrotechnic at 5 or 10 minute intervals. Once the green pyrotechnic has extinguished it should be answered immediately by the ignition of an answering red pyrotechnic from the distressed vessel or liferaft.

MAN OVERBOARD

Sometimes, although every precaution is taken, a person will fall overboard. In rough weather or at night they will quickly disappear from sight. An efficient method of location and recovery needs to be perfected by all crew members. Practising with a fender tied to a bucket as the 'man overboard' is a good exercise.

Immediately a person falls overboard, the following actions should be taken.

1 Shout **'Man Overboard'** to alert all the crew.

2 Throw in the dan buoy and a lifebelt.

3 Detail a crew member to observe and mark the position of the person in the water by pointing.

4 A buoyant orange smoke makes a good marker by day (see Pyrotechnics).

5 Immediately steer the propeller away from the casualty in the water by altering course towards the side over which he fell. Turn a tight circle until the boat is alongside or near the person overboard.

6 If necessary throw a line and when the person is secured to it, immediately put the engine in neutral.

7 Pull the victim in and secure alongside.

8 Use a ladder or scrambling net over the side of the boat for the casualty to climb back on board.

9 If necessary, form a loop tied with a fixed bowline knot in a rope and lower this over the person's body and pull him back on board.

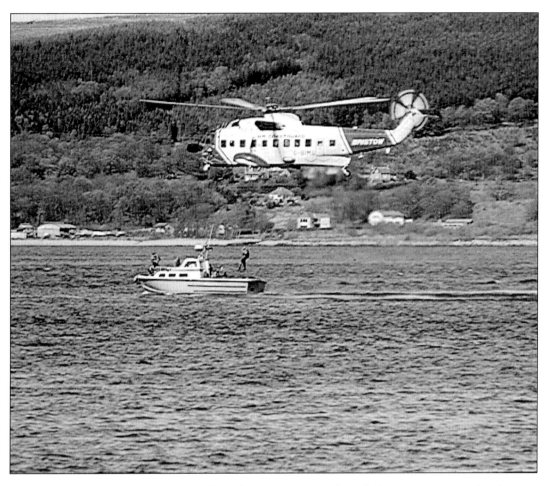

Helicopter pilots prefer to approach from the port quarter when the boat is motoring slowly into wind. Do not touch the winch wire until instructed. By courtesy of the Coastguard.

10 If the casualty is unconscious, someone has to go into the water. They must be attached to the boat by a strong line and have an inflated lifejacket.

11 When the person is brought alongside, if he is too heavy to lift out, it may be necessary to roll him into an inflated dinghy. If the boat has a tender secured with davits he can be raised in this. Another way is to place the person in the scrambling net, fold it like a bag, bringing the lower edge back on board, and haul in. If you have no net, lower a loop of rope to a rescuer in the water who passes it under the body (lying horizontally) and back up to helpers on the boat who can then haul up the victim; this is called parbuckling.

12 Rescuscitate if necessary (see Chapter 24) and treat for hypothermia and shock.

Note that a personal locator beacon considerable improves the chances of locating a person in the water. It is a small short-range beacon which is normally attached to a lifeacket. In conjunction with a direction-finder onboard, it provides a bearing from the boat to the man in the water.

MOTORMASTER

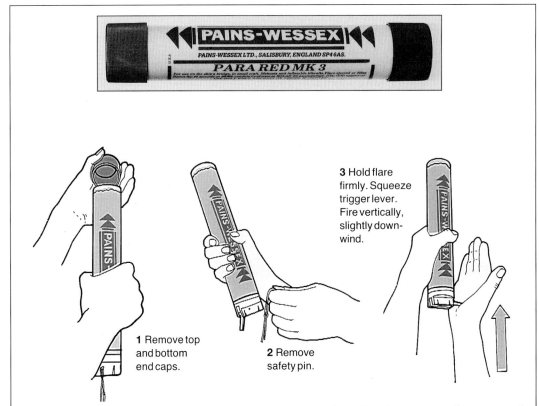

PAINS-WESSEX

PAINS-WESSEX LTD., SALISBURY, ENGLAND SP4 6AS.

PARA RED MK 3

3 Hold flare
firmly. Squeeze
trigger lever.
Fire vertically,
slightly down-
wind.

1 Remove top
and bottom
end caps.

2 Remove
safety pin.

Fig 22.1 *How to operate a hand-held red parachute rocket. This distress signal ejects a red flare suspended by a parachute at a height of 300 metres.*

Man Overboard lost from sight

In this situation, the only thing that can be done is to motor back on a reciprocal course through the area where the person was lost and then turn round and start a zigzag search pattern. A MAYDAY call should be initiated immediately on the VHF radio (see page 118).

PYROTECHNICS

Pyrotechnics are used to raise the alarm in a distress situation, pin-point the position when rescue is within sight and to warn another vessel of your position for collision avoidance and for illumination in a search situation.

Distress

Red flares and orange smoke signals are for use in a distress situation, when the boat or a member of the crew are in grave and imminent danger.

Red Parachute Rocket Flare

This is a hand-held signal ejecting a para-chute-suspended red flare to 300 m alti-tude. It burns for 40 seconds. It is a long range distress signal for use when 3 miles or more from land, but can be used when closer inshore than this if conditions war-rant. As a rocket turns into the wind it should normally be fired slightly down-wind to provide maximum range of visibil-ity. However, when there is low cloud, it is advisable to fire the rocket at an angle of

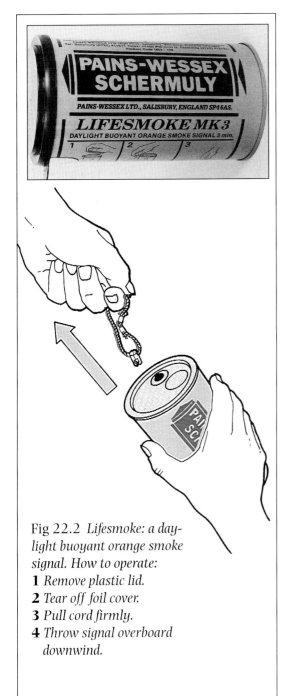

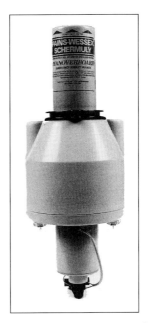

Man overboard marker or buoysmoke.

Fig 22.2 *Lifesmoke: a day-light buoyant orange smoke signal. How to operate:*
1 *Remove plastic lid.*
2 *Tear off foil cover.*
3 *Pull cord firmly.*
4 *Throw signal overboard downwind.*

45° in the direction from which help is most expected and so that it deploys below the cloud base.

Firing mechanisms are not all the same for different makes of flare so everyone on board should familiarise themselves with the mechanisms on pyrotechnics. The pyrotechnics described in this chapter are manufactured by Pains-Wessex Schermuly. Fig 22.1 shows how to fire a parachute flare.

Pinpointing position

To pin-point position once a rescue vessel is within sight, the following signals can be used:

Red handflare
This hand-held flare withstands extreme conditions and once ignited will continue to burn even during immersion. It burns for 60 seconds.

Handsmoke
A daylight distress signal. It produces dense orange smoke for 50 seconds and shows up well to aircraft.

Lifesmoke

This buoyant orange smoke signal consists of a metal canister fitted with a pull cord for ignition, (Fig 22.2). It burns for 3 minutes producing dense orange smoke and is safe to use on petrol or oil covered water.

Buoysmoke

An emergency smoke marker which can be mounted on deck and attached to the lifebuoy. It is stowed in the inverted position and automatically ignites when thrown in the water. It burns for 15 minutes producing dense orange smoke, and is safe to use on petrol or oil covered water. It is available combined with two lithium battery powered lights which burn for 2 hours and is specifically designed for man overboard situations (see photo on page 183).

Position Warning

A white handflare is used to draw attention to the boat's position when it is on a collision course with another vessel which does not appear to have seen it.

Emergency illumination

A white parachute rocket flare is very useful in an emergency search and rescue situation. It is projected to a height of 300 m and burns for 30 seconds.

Care of pyrotechnics

* Store in a secure dry place where they are easily accessible in an emergency.

* Make sure all the crew know their whereabouts and have read the operating instructions.

* Never use time expired pyrotechnics. These should be immediately replaced with new ones. Out of date pyrotechnics should be disposed of by the manufacturer or the Coastguard.

* Never point pyrotechnics at people.

* Should a signal fail to ignite, keep holding it in the firing position for at least 30 seconds. After this time, if it still has not ignited, remove the end caps so that water can penetrate and throw into the sea.

* Hold handflares and handsmokes downwind away from the boat and yourself so that burning particles fall in the water and smoke drifts away from the boat.

* Never look directly at handflares, they are very bright and can cause temporary blindness.

* Keep red and white flares separate so that they cannot be confused in the dark.

Recommended packs

Inshore – less than 3 miles from land
2 red handflares
2 orange handsmokes

Coastal – less than 7 miles from land
2 red handflares
2 orange handsmokes
2 red parachute rockets

Offshore – more than 7 miles from land
4 red handflares
4 red parachute rockets
2 lifesmokes

Collision avoidance
4 white handflares

Illumination
4 white parachute rockets

VHF RADIO

The quickest method of summoning help is to use the VHF radio; see Chapter 16.

TOWING AND SALVAGE

Towing

Towing or being towed occurs to most small craft at some time. The ideal arrangement is to use the towed vessel's anchor cable. A heaving line is passed between the two vessels to which the end of the towed vessel's anchor cable is attached and hauled inboard the towing vessel. On the towed vessel the inboard end of the anchor cable should be secured below deck with a rope lashing so that it can be slipped in an emergency. The advantage of using a chain cable is that the weight of the bight reduces snubbing (jerking), and, being strongly secured to the capstan or windlass, is not dependent upon a cleat on deck.

If it is not practical to use the anchor cable, then a heavy nylon warp should be used. Both on the towed and the towing vessel it is unlikely that the average cleat by itself will be strong enough for the snatch loads (suddenly applied loads) experienced during a tow. The load on any cleats used as towing points should be distributed by backing up either to other cleats or, if

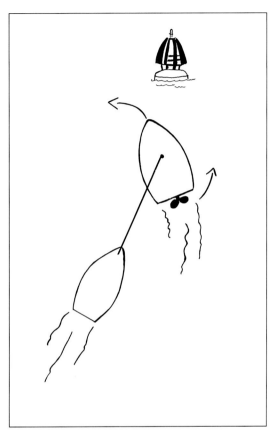

Fig 22.4 *When towing from astern, you will have better control if the tow is secured as centrally on your boat as possible.*

necessary, by a warp right around the superstructure or hull.

The towing situation can vary from quietly moving a vessel in harbour to pulling a vessel off a lee shore in heavy weather. In harbour it is usually easier to lash the two vessels alongside as shown in Fig 22.3.

At sea the most important consideration is to ensure that the vessel rendering assistance is not herself endangered, particularly by getting a rope around her propeller or running aground. When within a safe distance upwind of the vessel in difficulties, a line attached to a fender can be floated down. It may be prudent for the rescue vessel to drop her anchor in case she becomes unable to manoeuvre.

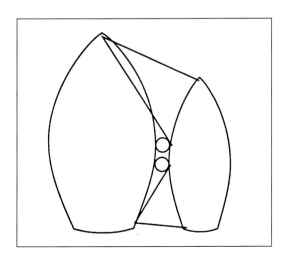

Fig 22.3 *Towing alongside.*

MOTORMASTER

Salvage

Towage is the amount payable to a tug or other vessel by agreement for towing a vessel anywhere.

Salvage is the voluntary act of saving or helping to save maritime property in danger. The following points should be born in mind when a tow is necessary:

- The RNLI never itself claims salvage or makes a charge. Lifeboatmen are legally entitled to claim salvage for themselves, but rarely do so.

- If a breakdown occurs in calm conditions always request a tow to a mutually agreed place and agree on a fee in advance.

- Unless in physical difficulties, do not allow any of the rescue vessel's crew to board your vessel.

- Never accept a tow line from the rescue vessel. Always pass your own tow line, steer your own vessel, give orders and have your anchor ready.

- Unless in distress, do not use distress signals to request assistance. Use VHF radio or hoist International Code flag 'V' (I require assistance).

- If salvage is claimed on the spot, endeavour to get an agreement in writing or have a witness to any discussion.

- If possible use the Lloyd's Open Form: Simple Form of Salvage Agreement 'No Cure – No Pay', obtainable from Salvage Arbritration Branch, Lloyd's of London, 1 Lime Street, London EC3M 7HA.

- Unless danger exists, no salvage claim can be made if the attempt is unsuccessful or if it results in the vessel getting into a worse position than she was in originally.

- If salvage is performed, always endeavour to produce a chart marked with the vessel's position and enter details, including weather conditions, in the deck log.

- If your vessel runs aground in a creek on a falling tide, never accept a 'pull off' from a stranger without saying that you are not in distress and do not need a tow. A friendly gesture can lead to a salvage claim. If you accept the loan of a heavy anchor and rope, make sure you agree a sum for its loan.

- If salvage is inevitable and a bargain unobtainable, never disclose the value of your vessel or insurance details.

QUESTIONS

22.1   a) When should a lifejacket be worn?
      b) When should a safety harness be worn?

22.2   What type of fire extinguisher should be used for:
      a) an electrical fire?
      b) an oil fire?

22.3   What is the correct action if a gas leak is suspected?

22.4   What is the recommended flare pack for:
      a) a boat on coastal passage not more than 5M from land?
      b) a boat on a cross channel passage?

22.5   Once you decide to use the liferaft, when should it be launched?

CHAPTER TWENTY THREE

COLLISION RULES & SIGNALS

THE INTERNATIONAL REGULATIONS FOR PREVENTING COLLISIONS AT SEA

Some of the rules particularly relevant to a motorboat are given here and explained.

Rule 5 – Lookout

Every vessel shall at all times maintain a proper look-out by sight and hearing as well as by all available means appropriate in the prevailing circumstances and conditions so as to make a full appraisal of the situation and of the risk of collision.

It is essential to keep a good lookout at all times. This means not only by looking and listening, but by using any means available such as radar. An effective lookout enables potentially hazardous situations to be observed in good time so that early and effective action can be taken.

On a motorboat with an enclosed steering position, parts of the boat may obstruct your view so it is essential to change position frequently so that you can view the whole horizon, or detail a crew member to do this. There is also loss of vision through spray and condensation on the windows and the noise from the engine masks engine noise and sound signals from other vessels. In conditions where there is poor visibility, if there is no outside steering position, it may be necessary to have an observer on deck.

Thoughtless use of cabin lights, torches and searchlights or matches can temporarily blind the helmsman and the lookout.

Rule 6 – Safe speed

Every vessel shall at all times proceed at a safe speed so that she can take proper and effective action to avoid collision and be stopped within a distance appropriate to the prevailing circumstances and conditions.

In determining a safe speed the following factors shall be among those taken into account:
(a) By all vessels:
(i) the state of visibility;
(ii) the traffic density including concentrations of fishing vessels or any other vessels;
(iii) the manoeuvrability of the vessel with special reference to stopping distance and turning ability in the prevailing conditions;
(iv) at night the presence of background light such as from shore lights or from back scatter of her own lights;
(v) the state of wind, sea and current, and the proximity of navigational hazards;
(vi) the draught in relation to the available depth of water.
(b) Additionally, by vessels with operational radar:
(i) the characteristics, efficiency and limitations of the radar equipment;
(ii) any constraints imposed by the radar range scale in use;
(iii) the effect on radar detection of the sea state, weather and other sources of interference;
(v) the number, location and movement of vessels detected by radar;
(vi) the more exact assessment of the visibility that may be possible when radar is used to determine the range of vessels or other objects in the vicinity.

A safe speed is determined by many things, the main ones being the volume of

MOTORMASTER

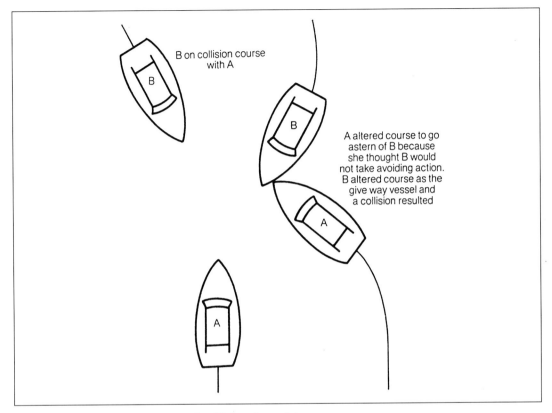

Fig 23.1 *Rule 8 – Action to avoid collision: how things can go wrong.*

traffic and visibility. The boat's manoeuvrability and stopping capability are important factors. A safe speed is one which gives plenty of time in the prevailing conditions to take safe and adequate action when necessary. Generally it can be thought of as being able to stop in half the distance you can see.

Rule 7 – Risk of collision

(a) Every vessel shall use all available means appropriate to the prevailing circumstances and conditions to determine if risk of collision exists. If there is any doubt such risk shall be deemed to exist.

(b) Proper use shall be made of radar equipment if fitted and operational, including long-range scanning to obtain early warning of risk of collision and radar plotting or equivalent systematic observation of detected objects.

(c) Assumptions shall not be made on the basis of scanty information, especially scanty radar information.

(d) In determining if risk of collision exists the following considerations shall be among those taken into account:

(i) such risk shall be deemed to exist if the compass bearing of an approaching vessel does not appreciably change;

(ii) such risk may sometimes exist even when an appreciable bearing change is evident, particularly when approaching a very large vessel or a tow or when approaching a vessel at close range.

If there is doubt about a risk of collision, then the risk is deemed to exist. To help to decide, a compass bearing of that vessel can be taken. This should be repeated at frequent intervals, say 1–2 minutes dependent upon the distance between vessels. If the bearing does not alter appreciably and the range decreases, then there is a risk of collision. (Fig 23.1).

Rule 8 – Action to avoid collision

(a) Any action taken to avoid collision shall, if the circumstances of the case admit, be positive, made in ample time and with due regard to the observance of good seamanship.

(b) Any alteration of course and/or speed to avoid collision shall, if the circumstances of the case admit, be large enough to be readily apparent to another vessel observing visually or by radar; a succession of small alterations of course and/or speed should be avoided.

(c) If there is sufficient sea room, alteration of course alone may be the most effective action to avoid a close-quarters situation provided that it is made in good time, is substantial and does not result in another close-quarters situation.

(d) Action taken to avoid collision with another vessel shall be such as to result in passing at a safe distance. The effectiveness of the action shall be carefully checked until the other vessel is finally past and clear.

(e) If necessary to avoid collision or allow more time to assess the situation, vessel shall slacken her speed or take all way off by stopping or reversing her means of propulsion.

(f)(i) A vessel which, by another of these rules, is required not to impede the passage or safe passage of another vessel shall, when required by the circumstances of the case, take early action to allow sufficient sea room for the safe passage of the other vessel;

(ii) A vessel required not to impede the passage or safe passage of another vessel is not relieved of this obligation if approaching the other vessel so as to involve risk of collision and shall, when taking action, have full regard to the action which may be required by the rules of this part.

(iii) A vessel the passage of which is not to be impeded remains fully obliged to comply with the rules of this part when the two vessels are approaching one another so as to involve risk of collision.

Any action taken to avoid collision needs to be *positive, early* and *obvious* enough to be recognised by the other vessel. A small alteration to course or speed to avoid a collision may not be immediately obvious to the other vessel and can cause confusion. A positive action such as presenting a different aspect to the other vessel, particularly at night, is much better and safer. A considerable reduction of speed will give the situation time to change and the helmsman time to sort out a more complicated situation in congested waters.

You should take action early. If you leave it until the last minute the other vessel will be confused and may assume that no action is going to be taken. If it then alters course at the same time as you do, a collision could ensue, Fig 23.1.

Avoid crossing the bows of another vessel to which you are giving way until well clear.

Rule 10 – Traffic separation schemes

(a) This Rule applies to traffic separation schemes adopted by the Organisation and does not relieve any vessel of her obligation under any other rule.

(b) A vessel using a traffic separation scheme shall:

(i) proceed in the appropriate traffic lane in the general direction of traffic flow for that lane;

(ii) so far as practicable keep clear of a traffic separation line or separation zone;

(iii) normally join or leave a traffic lane at the termination of the lane, but when joining or leaving from either side shall do so at as small an angle to the general direction of traffic flow as practicable.

(c) A vessel shall, so far as practicable, avoid crossing traffic lanes, but if obliged to do so shall cross on a heading as nearly as practicable at right angles to the general direction of traffic flow.

(d) Inshore traffic zones shall not normally be used by through traffic which can safely use the appropriate traffic lane within the adjacent traffic separation scheme. However, vessels of less than 20 metres in length and sailing vessels may under all circumstances use inshore traffic zones.

(e) A vessel other than a crossing vessel or a vessel joining or leaving a lane shall not normally enter a separation zone or cross a separation line except:
 (i) in case of emergency to avoid immediate danger;
 (ii) to engage in fishing within a separation zone.

(f) A vessel navigating in areas near the terminations of traffic separation schemes shall do so with particular caution.

(g) A vessel shall so far as practicable avoid anchoring in a traffic separation scheme or in areas near its terminations.

(h) A vessel not using a traffic separation scheme shall avoid it by as wide a margin as is practicable.

(i) A vessel engaged in fishing shall not impede the passage of any vessel following a traffic lane.

(j) A vessel of less than 20 metres in length or a sailing vessel shall not impede the safe passage of a power-driven vessel following a traffic lane.

(k) A vessel restricted in her ability to manoeuvre when engaged in an operation for the maintenace of safety of navigation in a traffic separation scheme is exempted from complying with this Rule to the extent necessary to carry out the operation.

(l) A vessel restricted in her ability to manoeuvre when engaged in an operation for the laying, servicing or picking up of a submarine cable, within a traffic separation scheme, is exempted from complying with the Rule to the extent necessary to carry out the operation.

The Traffic Separation Scheme is marked on charts by a series of large arrows. It consists of two one-way traffic lanes separated by a separation zone. These lanes are used by larger vessels. If possible, the Traffic Separation Scheme should be avoided. However, if obliged to cross it then the boat's *heading* must be at right angles to the traffic lanes. This presents a 90° aspect to lane users, which may not be the case if the boat's *track* were at right angles to the traffic lane.

A boat of less than 20 m in length should not impede the passage of a vessel using the traffic lane. This conflicts with Rule 15. It is, however, common sense for small craft to avoid larger ones by taking early action in areas where there is high traffic density.

Rule 13 – Overtaking

(a) Notwithstanding anything contained in the Rules of Part B, Sections 1 and 2, any vessel overtaking any other shall keep out of the way of the vessel being overtaken.

(b) A vessel shall be deemed to be overtaking when coming up with another vessel from a direction more than 22.5 degrees abaft her beam, that is, in such a position with reference to the vessel she is overtaking, that at night she would be able to see only the sternlight of that vessel but neither of her sidelights.

(c) When a vessel is in any doubt as to whether she is overtaking another, she shall assume that this is the case and act accordingly.

(d) Any subsequent alteration of the bearing between the two vessels shall not make the overtaking vessel a crossing vessel within the meaning of these Rules of relieve her of the duty of keeping clear of the overtaken vessel until she is finally past and clear.

An overtaking vessel must keep clear of the boat being overtaken. The overtaken boat must not impede the overtaking vessel.

Rule 14 – Head-on situation

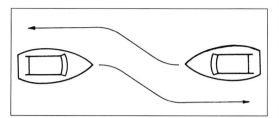

Fig 23.2 *Rule 14 states that power-driven vessels meeting head-on shall both turn to starboard.*

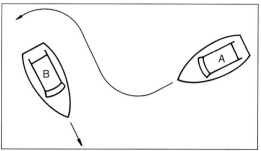

Fig 23.3 *In this situation, Rule 15 requires A to turn to starboard to go astern of B.*

(a) When two power-driven vessels are meeting on reciprocal or nearly reciprocal courses so as to involve risk of collision each shall alter her course to starboard so that each shall pass on the port side of the other.

(b) Such a situation shall be deemed to exist when a vessel sees the other ahead or nearly ahead and by night she could see the masthead lights of the other in a line or nearly in a line and/or both side-lights and by day she observes the corresponding aspect of the other vessel.

(c) When a vessel is in any doubt as to whether such a situation exists she shall assume that it does exist and act accordingly.

SIGNALS USED WHEN VESSELS ARE IN SIGHT OF ONE ANOTHER

●	One short blast	I am altering course to starboard.
●●	Two short blasts	I am altering course to port.
●●●	Three short blasts	My engines are going astern.
●●●●●	Five short blasts	I am unsure of your intentions.
●●●● ●	Four short blasts followed by one short blast	I intend to turn completely around to starboard.
●●●● ●●	Four short blasts followed by two short blasts	I intend to turn completely around to port.
■■ ●	Two long blasts followed by one short blast	I wish to overtake you on your starboard side.
■■ ●●	Two long blasts followed by two short blasts	I wish to overtake you on your port side.
■●■●	One long blast, one short blast, one long blast, one short blast	You may overtake me on the side indicated.

MOTORMASTER

If two vessels meet on reciprocal courses with a risk of collision, each shall alter course to starboard so that each shall pass on the port side of the other, ie red to red.

Rule 15 – Crossing situation

When two power-driven vessels are crossing so as to involve risk of collision, the vessel which has the other on her own starboard side shall keep out of the way and shall, if the circumstances of the case admit, avoid crossing ahead of the other vessel.

The correct action in a crossing situation is for the vessel who sees the *other* vessel to starboard to keep clear and if necessary, to alter course to starboard and pass astern of the other vessel. Fig 23.3.

Rule 18 – Responsibilities between vessels

Except where Rules 9, 10 and 13 otherwise require:

(a) A power-driven vessel underway shall keep out of the way of:

(i) a vessel not under command;

(ii) a vessel restricted in her ability to manoeuvre;

(iii) a vessel engaged in fishing;

(iv) a sailing vessel;

(b) A sailing vessel underway shall keep out of the way of:

(i) a vessel not under command;

(ii) a vessel restricted in her ability to manoeuvre;

(iii) a vessel engaged in fishing.

(c) A vessel engaged in fishing when underway shall as far as possible, keep out of the way of:

(i) A vessel not under command;

(ii) a vessel restricted in her ability to manoeuvre;

(d) (i) Any vessel other than a vessel not under command or a vessel restricted in her ability to manoeuvre shall, if the cirucmstances of the case admit, avoid impeding the safe passage of a vessel contrained by her draught, exhibiting the signals in Rule 28.

(ii) A vessel constrained by her draft shall navigate with particular caution having full regard to her special condition.

(e) A seaplane on the water shall, in general, keep well clear of all vessels and avoid impeding their navigation. In circumstances, however, where risk of collision exists, she shall comply with the Rules of this Part.

Rule 19 – Conduct of vessels in restricted visibility

(a) This Rule applies to vessels not in sight of one another when navigating in or near an area of restricted visibility.

(b) Every vessel shall proceed at a safe speed adapted to the prevailing circumstances and conditions of restricted visibility. A power-driven vessel shall have her engines ready for immediate manoeuvre.

(c) Every vessel shall have due regard to the prevailing circumstances and conditions of restricted visibility when complying with the Rules of Section 1 of this Part.

(d) A vessel which detects by radar alone the presence of another vessel shall determine if a close-quarters situation is developing and/or risk of collision exists. If so, she shall take avoiding action in ample time, provided that when such action consists of an alteration of course, so far as possible the following shall be avoided:

(i) an alteration of course to port for a vessel forward of the beam, other than for a vessel being overtaken;

(ii) an alteration of course towards a vessel abeam or abaft the beam.

(e) Except where it has been determind that a risk of collision does not exist, every vessel which hears apparently foward of her beam the fog signal of another vessel, or which cannot avoid a close-quarters situation with another vessel forward of her beam, shall reduce her speed to the minimum at which she can be kept on her course. She shall if necessary take all her way off and in any event navigate with extreme caution until danger of collision is over.

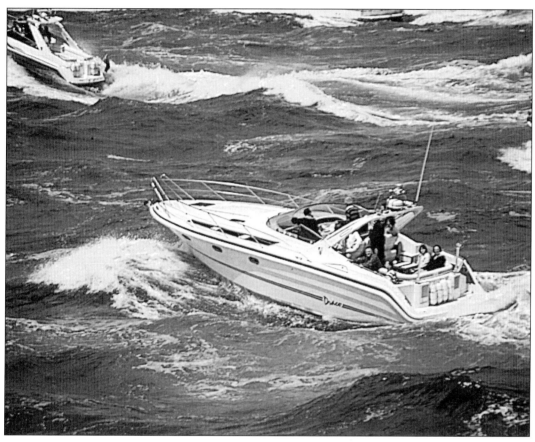

According to the IRPCS rules, an overtaking vessel must keep clear of the boat being overtaken; in rough water leave plenty of space between vessels.

Extra care is needed in conditions where visibility is reduced and you need to keep to a safe speed. The boat must keep a constant lookout by sight and sound with a crew member on deck at the bows away from engine noise to listen for other vessels and their fog signals. An efficient radar reflector must be hoisted if one is not permanently fixed. If in a Traffic Separation Scheme it is best to leave it by the fastest route and keep well clear until visibility improves. Moving into shallower water where large vessels are unlikely to pass is a good option. The boat should be ready to manoeuvre immediately and take sub-stantial action where necessary to avoid collision.

Rule 34 – Manoeuvring and Warning signals

See page 191.

Rule 35 – Sound signals in restricted visibility

See page 194.

MOTORMASTER

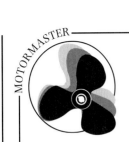
LIGHTS, SHAPES AND FOG SIGNALS

Below are given the light configurations needed at night by various vessels together with the day shapes and fog sound signals.

The letters in circles represent the colours of the lights and their positions on the vessel in question: Green, Red and White. The directional aspect of the boat is given underneath the diagram ie bow: the bow of the vessel is being viewed so you would expect to see the port hand (red) light on the right and the starboard hand (green) light on the left.

The shapes given are those which are obliged to be displayed by vessels carrying out certain manoeuvres.

RULE 23 Power driven vessel under way less than 50 metres in length			
ⓌⒼ Ⓡ Bow	Ⓦ Ⓡ View from Port	Ⓦ Stern	▬ Fog sound signal One long blast
RULE 24 Towing vessel - tow more than 200 metres long			
Ⓦ Ⓦ Ⓦ Ⓖ Ⓡ Bow	Ⓦ Ⓦ Ⓦ Ⓖ View from Stbd	Ⓨ Ⓦ Stern	◆ DAY SHAPE Tug ▬ ●● Tow ▬ ●●● Fog sound signal
RULE 25 Sailing vessel underway			
Ⓖ◖Ⓡ less than 20m ⒼⓇ over 20m Under sail Bow	Ⓦ Ⓖ Ⓡ Under power Bow	Ⓦ Stern	▬ ●● Under sail ▬ Under power Fog sound signal

Note: Sailing vessels may carry a tricolour light at the masthead.

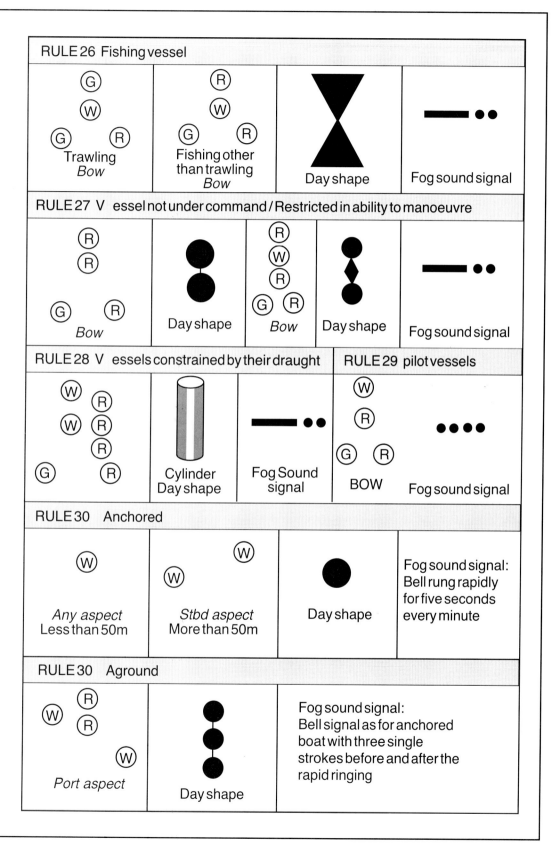

RULE 26 Fishing vessel

G / W / G / R
Trawling
Bow

R / W / G / R
Fishing other than trawling
Bow

Day shape

Fog sound signal

RULE 27 Vessel not under command / Restricted in ability to manoeuvre

R / R / G / R
Bow

Day shape

R / W / R / G / R
Bow

Day shape

Fog sound signal

RULE 28 Vessels constrained by their draught

W / R / W / R / R / G / R

Cylinder Day shape

Fog Sound signal

RULE 29 pilot vessels

W / R / G / R
BOW

Fog sound signal

RULE 30 Anchored

W
Any aspect Less than 50m

W / W
Stbd aspect More than 50m

Day shape

Fog sound signal: Bell rung rapidly for five seconds every minute

RULE 30 Aground

W / R / R / W
Port aspect

Day shape

Fog sound signal: Bell signal as for anchored boat with three single strokes before and after the rapid ringing

MOTORMASTER

195

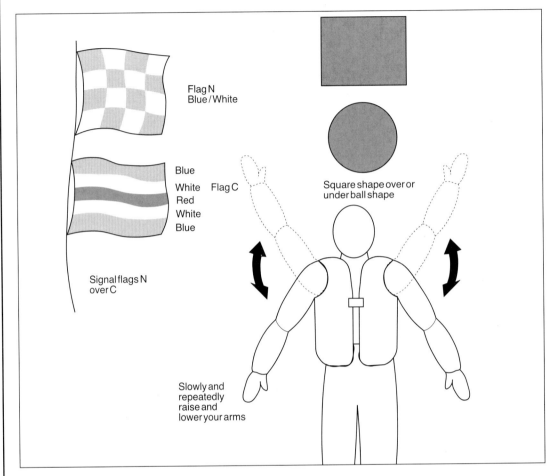

Fig 23.4 *Some distress signals.*

Distress Signals

The international distress signals are listed in Annex IV of the Collision Regulations. Some are intended for use by larger commercial vessels only.

The following are the distress signals particularly applicable to smaller motor vessels.

- Continuous sounding with any fog signalling apparatus

- SOS by any method

- Mayday by VHF radio

- International Code flags N over C, (Fig 23.4)

- Square flag above or below a ball, (Fig 23.4)

- Red rocket parachute flare

- Orange smoke signal

- Slowly and repeatedly raising and lowering arms (Fig 23.4)

- Signal transmitted from Emergency Position Indicating Radio Beacon (EPIRB).

All distress signals are for the purpose of indicating distress and the need for assistance and should not be used for other purposes. The use of signals which may be confused with distress signals is prohibited.

MOTORMASTER

QUESTIONS

23.1 What are the main factors to determine a safe speed?

23.2 How can you determine whether a risk of collision exists when in sight of an approaching vessel?

23.3 What do the following sound signals mean? (Fig 23.5). State whether they are manoeuvring and warning signals or signals made in restricted visibility.

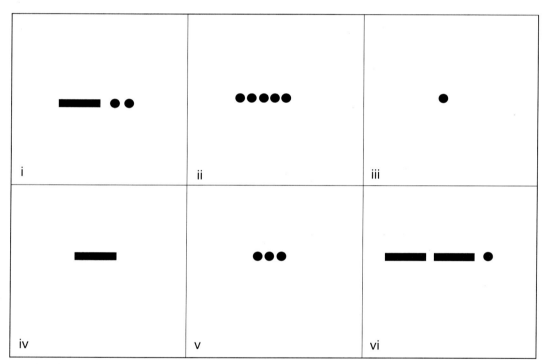

Fig 23.5

23.4 In Fig 23.6 (page 198), which vessel is required to give way?

23.5 In Fig 23.7 (page 198), what type of vessel is it, is it underway, and which aspect is presented?

23.6 When a collision situation exists, what action should you take to avoid collision?

23.7 If it is necessary to cross a Traffic Separation Scheme, how should this be done?

23.8 When should a lookout be kept?

23.9 Give five distress signals suitable for a 10 m motorboat.

MOTORMASTER

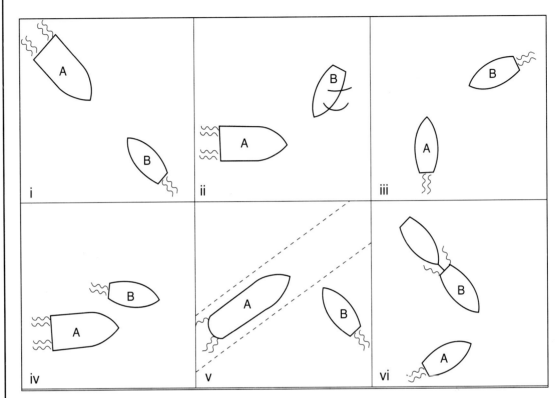

Fig 23.6.

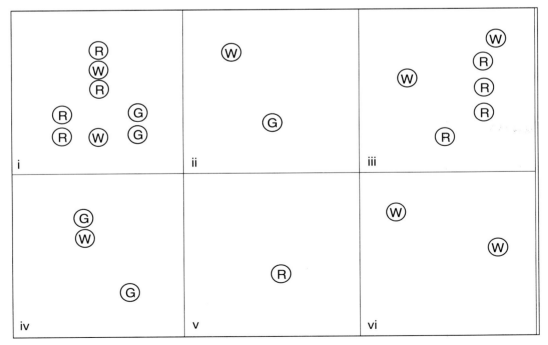

Fig 23.7.

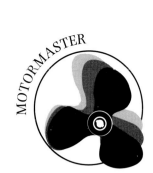

CHAPTER TWENTY FOUR

FIRST AID

First aid is the first help or treatment administered to a casualty whilst awaiting the arrival of a qualified medical authority. The aim of first aid is to:

- Preserve life.

- Stop the condition worsening.

- Help promote recovery.

Following an accident at sea it may be some time before assistance arrives and any casualty can be taken ashore, so any action taken must be quick, correct and thorough. It is essential therefore, that all boat users have a sound knowledge of what to do in these circumstances. Such a knowledge can be gained by attending an approved first aid course. It is also vital to know how to summon help.

If you are out at sea, contacting the Coastgbuard by VHF radio is your best course of action, so you should regard a radio as an essential piece of emergency equipment. If you fear that the casualty is gravely ill then send out a MAYDAY call which will receive immediate priority; if your casualty is injured or unwell but is not seriously ill then send a PAN PAN MEDICO call (See Chapter 16).

You must be aware of any medication taken by other crew members and of any conditions which may require special treatment.

In all but minor accidents, treatment for shock should be given. The casualty should be watched in case he or she becomes unconscious and breathing and heart stop; and should then be referred to a doctor as soon as possible. Any person who has had their lungs full of water (apparently drowned) must be referred to hospital as soon as possible even if they seem to have recovered as they may later suffer from secondary drowning when the lungs refill with fluid.

INCIDENT MANAGEMENT

It is important in an emergency, that one person takes charge and assumes responsibility for incident management. They should ideally have a basic knowledge of first aid and be able to respond quickly and make a rapid assessment of the situation. They should be able to direct others on the scene to summon help, fetch equipment, carry out resuscitation or whatever aid is needed.

The incident manager should monitor and evaluate the condition of the victim and be able to make decisions as to the best course of action. The following points are important for your evaluation:

- Is the patient conscious or unconscious?

- Does he or she need to be removed from further danger?

- Are there people close at hand who can render assistance or summon help?

- Are the helpers themselves likely to be in danger (it is essential to avoid further casualties)?

- Do you have first aid equipment to hand? If not, can you improvise?

- Are there any other persons involved in the incident who may need attention? It is all too easy to focus all attention on the most seriously affected victim – there may be others who need your care.

Remember, for effective aid you need to assess the situation, make a plan and act promptly:

ASSESS – PLAN – ACT

A—Z OF FIRST AID TREATMENT

BLEEDING (SEVERE)

Treatment

1 The casualty should be laid down.

2 Pressure should be applied directly to the wound using a pad of sterile material (if this is available) or a towel or clothing. If there is nothing else then use your hand. Squeeze gaping wounds together.

3 Secure the pad firmly with a bandage, if you have one, to maintain the pressure.

4 Should the wound bleed through the initial dressing, a further one should be applied over the top of it. Keep the patient still.

5 For arm and leg wounds, the limb can be elevated.

6 If wounds to the limbs cannot be controlled by local pressure and elevation, indirect pressure can be used. This is done by pressing an artery against a bone. This method should only be used when all else has failed and bleeding is severe, as it cuts off the blood supply to the whole limb. The pressure must not be applied for more than 15 minutes, otherwise serious damage will be caused to the limb.

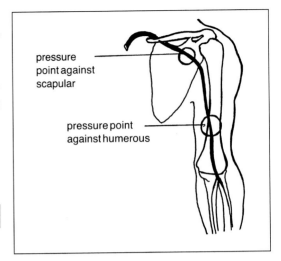

Fig 24.1 *Pressure points on the brachial artery in the upper arm.*

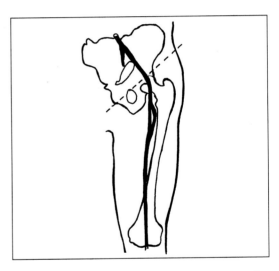

Fig 24.2 *Pressure point (dotted line) on the femoral artery in the groin.*

There are two pressure points concerned, the brachial artery which is on the inner side of the upper arm, Fig 24.1, and the femoral artery which is at the centre of the groin, Fig 24.2. Pressure is applied with the fingers.

MOTORMASTER

BURNS AND SCALDS

Treatment

1 Immediately immerse the affected part in cold water to cool the area and prevent further burning. If this is not possible, pour cold seawater over the area. This should be done for at least 10 minutes.

2 As the area will swell, remove anything likely to constrict the circulation, such as bracelets, watches, rings or shoes.

3 Cut away any loose clothing but leave any adhering to the wound.

4 Cover with a non fluffy sterile dressing or cling film.

5 Treat for shock (see page 224).

6 Keep the patient warm and give plenty of water to drink.

7 In all but minor cases seek medical help.

Chemical burns

Treatment

1 Pour cold water over the area for at least 10 minutes to stop the chemical doing further damage.

2 Remove any contaminated clothing but take care not to burn your hands.

3 Cover the area with a non fluffy sterile dressing or cling film.

4 Treat for shock (see page 210).

5 If severe, seek medical help.

CHEST INJURY

Fractured ribs – signs:

- Pain in the chest.
- Difficult breathing.
- Rib cage may have lost its rigidity.
- Tenderness over the fracture.
- Bloodstained sputum may be coughed up indicating damage to the lung.

Treatment

1 Get the casualty into a semi-sitting position inclined towards the injured side.

2 Fold a newspaper or pad of stiff material and place over the injury. Put the casualty's arm over this across the chest with the fingers pointing to the opposite shoulder. Secure with a sling or bandage.

3 Encourage the casualty to move as little as possible as there is a danger of a broken rib penetrating a lung.

Penetrating wound – signs:

- Pain at and around the site of the injury.
- Difficult breathing.
- Lips and nail bed may be blue.
- Blood may be coughed up and also ooze from the wound.
- There may be a sucking noise from the wound as the casualty breathes in.

Treatment

1 The wound must be sealed immediately to stop the lung collapsing. An airtight dressing should be placed on it made from a sterile pad over which is taped a piece of plastic or metal foil.

2 Do not attempt to remove the object if it is still in the wound as this may aggravate the condition.

3 Place in a semi-sitting position inclined towards the injured side.

MOTORMASTER

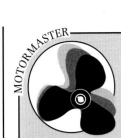

RESUSCITATION

If the casualty has stopped breathing artifical ventilation will be required. Check the pulse in the carotid artery on the front left of the neck. If there is no heartbeat, cardiac compression must be administered without delay.

NOT BREATHING BUT HEART BEATING

1 Lie the casualty face upwards on a hard surface. Loosen tight clothing round the neck.

2 See that there is an open airway. Clear the mouth of debris or anything likely to cause a blockage. Remove dentures.

3 Carefully push the head back as far as it will go and at the same time pull the chin upwards and forwards to achieve a good neck extension. This action will keep the tongue clear of the back of the throat and maintain an open airway. The casualty may start to breathe after this is done, Fig 24.3.

4 If breathing does not start, keep the head in the tilted position, pinch the nose to seal it, take a deep breath, seal your lips around the casualty's mouth and breath into the lungs. The chest should rise.

5 The air should be allowed to escape naturally, and whilst this is happening, turn your face away from the casualty's, take another deep breath and again breath into the casualty's lungs.

6 The first 6 inflations should be given as quickly as possible, thereafter repeating at the normal breathing rate until the casualty is breathing normally. Once you have begun artificial ventilation it is your obligation to *continue until a qualified medical practitioner can take over care of the patient.*

7 On resuming breathing, the victim will probably vomit so should not be left unattended at any time. When normal breathing has been resumed, unless there are injuries which prevent it, place the casualty in the recovery position (see Fig 24.7), under supervision, as breathing may cease again.

8 If for any reason mouth to mouth respiration cannot be carried out, the mouth can be sealed by using your thumb, and mouth to nose respiration performed.

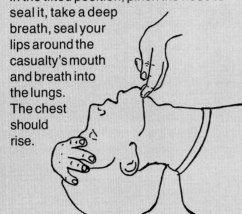

Fig 24.3 *Before starting artificial ventilation, extend the neck by lifting the chin and pushing the forehead back. Do not obstruct the throat. Check the mouth for loose dentures or food.*

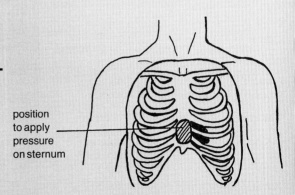

position to apply pressure on sternum

Fig 24.5 *This shows the part of the sternum (breast bone) where the pressure should be applied for cardiac compressions.*

Children

For a child, your lips can seal both mouth and nose. The ventilations should be given gently, about 20 breaths a minute.

In-water casualty

Artificial ventilation can be performed while you are supporting a casualty in the water and he or she stops breathing. Check the mouth for obstructions and clear the airway. Extend the neck and hold the jaws shut, tilted upwards. Take a good breath and seal your lips over the nose. Blow into the nose, repeating ventilations until the victim can be recovered into the boat. Remember – act fast and positively, seconds count.

NOT BREATHING WITH HEART STOPPED

If no heartbeat can be found by listening at the chest or by checking the carotid pulse in the neck, the heart has stopped and chest compression must be administered immediately.

1 Lie the casualty on a hard surface.

2 The heart is stimulated by pressure on the breastbone – locate the lower end and apply the heel of the palm on the lower half of the breastbone. Position the hands as shown in Fig 24.5. Keep the arms straight and do not let the elbows bend.

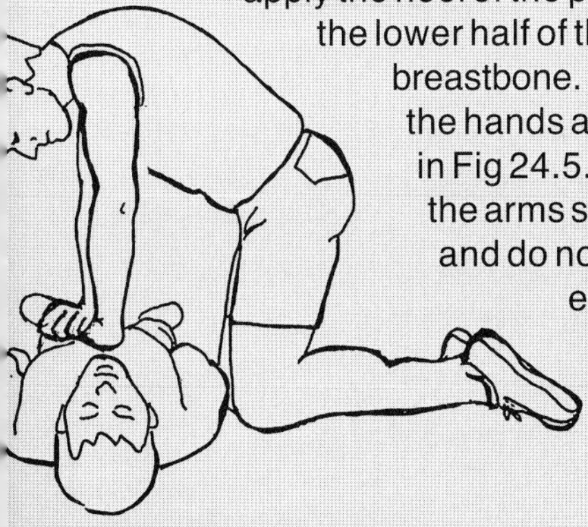

Fig 24.6 While leaning over the casualty, apply the heel of one hand to the position shown in Fig 24.5. Cover this hand with the heel of the other and apply pressure firmly with straight arms. Release the pressure and repeat at a rate of about 80 per minute.

3 Press downwards, using your body weight transmitted through straight arms. The pressure should be sufficient to compress the chest 4–5 cm (1½–2 in). The rate should be about 80 per minute.

4 Artificial ventilation must be combined with cardiac compressions, giving 15 compressions to 2 ventilations.

5 The carotid pulse in the neck should be checked after the first minute and then every 3 minutes. As soon as the heart is beating, compression is stopped, but artificial ventilation continues until breathing is normal. It is vital not to continue compressions after the heart has restarted as they could cause it to stop again.

6 When the heart is beating and breathing is normal, the casualty should be placed in the recovery position (Fig 24.7) and watched.

Children

A light pressure only using the heel of the hand is given to children. For babies the pressure of two fingers is sufficient. The rate for children and babies is about 100 per minute.

RECOVERY POSITION

An unconscious person whose heart is beating, and who is breathing normally, should be placed in the recovery position, as this will stop the tongue falling back into the throat and blocking the airway. It will also drain vomit from the mouth which might otherwise choke the casualty.

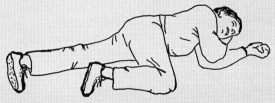

Fig 24.7 The recovery position. Make sure that there is a good neck extension for breathing and that the head is tilted to allow any vomit to flow away from the face.

CHOKING

This is caused by something blocking the airway to the lungs.

Treatment

1 Remove dentures. Try to dislodge the object by encouraging the casualty to cough.

2 If this fails, sit the casualty down and bend them forwards so that the head is lower than the lungs. Administer a series of slaps between the shoulder blades using the heel of the hand. A child can be bent over the knee and a baby held upside-down to do this.

3 If the object is still not dislodged, stand behind the casualty with your arms around their abdomen just below the ribs, clench one fist with your thumb inwards and grasp it with the other hand. Squeeze the casualty as tightly as possible using a quick upward thrust to compress the abdomen. This should move the obstruction. Repeat as necessary. This method should be used only after other methods have failed as damage can be caused.

As soon as possible the casualty should be examined by a doctor to see that no internal injury has been caused.

CORAL GRAZE

This may later become infected and need medical treatment.

Treatment

1 Clean with antiseptic.

2 Apply a sterile dressing.

CUTS

Unless deep or large, allow to bleed for a short time as this helps to cleanse the wound. Wash with a little antiseptic and cover with a sterile dressing. Cuts constantly exposed to seawater will not heal quickly.

For deep cuts, if the casualty has not had a tetanus injection within the last ten years, they should see a doctor.

DISLOCATIONS AND FRACTURES

Treatment

1 Immobilise the injured area in the most comfortable position.

2 If splints are used the ties are placed above and below the site of the injury. These must not be too tight or they will stop the circulation especially if the limb swells.

3 Padding is required between legs and between arm and body.

4 Inflatable splints are useful but do not overinflate so as to constrict circulation.

5 The extremities should be inspected regularly to see that they are not becoming blue. If they are, the bindings are too tight and must be loosened off.

6 If possible elevate an injured limb.

7 Spinal injuries must be kept as still as possible to prevent further damage.

FISH HOOK

Treatment

If the hook is not in very far it can be eased

out. When it is firmly embedded, a different technique has to be used.

1 Cut the line.

2 Grasp the hook firmly using pliers if necessary and push through the flesh until the barb appears, Fig 24.8a.

3 Cut the barb off near the flesh using the pliers, Fig 24.8b.

4 Withdraw the shank, Fig 24.8c.

5 Clean the wound and cover with a dressing.

6 If the wound becomes infected seek medical help. A tetanus injection may be needed.

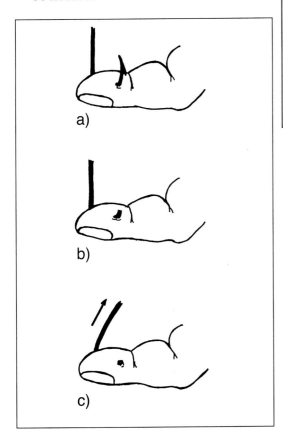

Fig 24.8 *How to remove a fish hook:*
a) push hook through until barb is exposed;
b) cut off barb; c) withdraw shank.

FIRST AID KIT

A Brook airway is an inexpensive aid for resuscitation but it should be used with care.

Adhesive elastic strapping
Adhesive suture strips
Adhesive waterproof dressings
Antiseptic wipes
Antiseptic
Adhesive plasters
Bandages
Calamine lotion
Constipation tablets
Cottonwool
Crepe bandage
Diarrhoea tablets
Exposure bag
Eyebath, eye lotion and eyepad
Finger stalls

First aid manual
Gauze burn dressing
Gauze swabs
Indigestion tablets
Pain relief tablets
Plastic skin
Safety pins
Scissors
Seasickness tablets
Sunscreen
Thermometer
Triangular bandages
Tweezers
Wound dressings, various sizes
Vaseline

Improvised First Aid Materials

There are many items around the boat which can be used in case of emergency.

Splints
Oars from the dinghy, if available, and floorboards can be used.

Bandages
Any clean material such as a pillow case or handkerchief.

Slings
Pillowcase, tea towel, belt.

Pads
Tea towel, towel.

Stretcher

Two jackets can be buttoned up and dinghy oars pushed through the sleeves; the sides of a large blanket can be rolled around the oars; or a cabin door can be used.

Cooling

Remember that the boat is surrounded by cold or cool seawater, ideal for applying to burns, scalds, and for heatstroke.

FOREIGN BODY IN THE EYE

Treatment

1 Do not let the casualty rub the eye.

2 Ask them to pull the upper lid over the lower one and roll the eye around.

3 If this does not work, sit them down with their head back and stand behind.

4 Separate the lids by using the thumb and first finger and ask them to roll their eye around so that you can inspect all parts of it.

5 If the foreign body can be seen and it is not adhering to the eye, it can gently be removed with a damp cotton bud or the corner of a clean damp handkerchief.

6 Alternatively an eye bath can be used to wash the object out or the casualty can immerse the eye in a bowl of water and blink. If this is not possible, a jug of water can be poured over the eye with the casualty's head inclined to the injured side. If any chemicals are involved constantly rinse the eye with water.

7 If the foreign body cannot be removed, cover with a sterile pad and seek medical help.

HEADACHE

Headaches are often caused by sunlight especially if it is reflecting off the water. Protective sunglasses should always be worn. Aspirin or paracetamol may help. If severe, the casualty should lie down in a cool place with a cold compress over the eyes.

If persistent it may be a symptom of a more serious condition such as heatstroke.

HEAD WOUNDS

After a blow on the head the brain can become disturbed or damaged. Consciousness may be lost or clouded and concussion or brain compression may occur. The casualty may become drowsy or go into a coma. All bumps on the head should be referred to a doctor.

Concussion

Signs

• Brief or slight loss of consciousness.

• Shallow breathing.

• Pallor.

• Skin cold and clammy.

• Rapid and weak pulse.

• As the casualty recovers they may vomit.

• Upon recovering the casualty may not recollect any event just prior to the accident and may be generally confused. Ask the casualty if they know the date, the time and their location.

Treatment

1 If the casualty has apparently recovered, make comfortable and frequently check

to see that their condition is not deteriorating. Rest and regular observation should continue for 24 hours.

2 If the casualty is unconscious and cannot be roused by calling their name and shaking, place in the recovery position (provided that there are no injuries to prevent this) so that the casualty does not inhale vomit. Should the person not return to consciousness, treat for compression.

Compression

Compression occurs due to a damaged brain swelling, fluid accumulation, or bone pressure from a depressed fracture. This is a serious condition from which the casualty can die. They need urgent medical assistance. The symptoms can become evident some time after apparent recovery which is why a casualty who has suffered any head injury should be monitored and referred to a doctor as soon as possible.

Signs

• Level of responsiveness lessens.

• Noisy breathing.

• Slow but strong pulse.

• Pupils of unequal size.

• Temperature may rise.

• Face may become flushed but remain dry.

Treatment

1 Loosen clothing.

2 Dress any wounds and place the patient in the recovery position.

3 Treat for shock.

4 Unconsciousness can happen several hours after the accident so the casualty should be watched to see that breathing and heart do not stop. Check and keep a record of responsiveness, breathing and pulse rate every 10 minutes.

5 Note time of injury and length of any period of unconsciousness.

6 Ensure airway unobstructed as vomiting very likely.

7 Arrange for removal to hospital as quickly as possible.

HEART ATTACK

Signs

• Severe pain in the centre of the chest radiating out to the arms, neck, back and abdomen.

• Dizziness and breathlessness.

• Pale skin and blue lips.

• Perspiring.

• Pulse fast and irregular.

• May become unconscious and breathing and heart stop.

Treatment

Reassure the casualty, make them comfortable and see that they do not put any extra strain on their heart by moving around.

1 Loosen tight clothing.

2 Place in a sitting position, knees bent.

3 Be ready to resuscitate if breathing and heart stop.

4 Summon immediate help by VHF radio if possible.

MOTORMASTER

HEAT EXHAUSTION

When the body temperature rises during exercise, fluid and salt are lost during perspiration. If the environment is hot and moist and the body fluids are not replaced, heat exhaustion can occur.

Signs

- Feeling exhausted.
- Headache and fainting.
- Muscular cramps.
- Breathing quick and shallow.
- Pulse weak and rapid.
- Temperature falls or remains normal.

Treatment

1 Lie the casualty in a cool place and let them sip cold water to which salt has been added (half a teaspoonful to half a litre of water).

2 If the casualty becomes unconscious, place in the recovery position and watch that breathing does not stop.

HEAT STROKE

This is caused by exposure to heat and high humidity for too long a period, when the body becomes unable to regulate the temperature by perspiration.

Signs

- Feeling hot.
- Headache.
- High temperature.
- Perspiring.

- Vomiting and dizziness.
- Collapse and unconsciousness.

Treatment

1 Lower the casualty's body temperature immediately by stripping off their clothing, wrap in a sheet and dowse with buckets of seawater until thoroughly saturated.

2 Sit the casualty in the shade in a draught. (It may be necessary to motor to create a draught.)

3 Keep wet and in a draught until their temperature falls.

4 If the casualty becomes unconscious place in the recovery position and monitor breathing.

5 When the temperature returns to normal, place in a cool shady position and check the temperature regularly. If it rises again, repeat the above procedure.

HYPOTHERMIA

Hypothermia is a severe cooling of the inner core which, if not halted, can cause death in a short while. It is caused by continuous exposure to a cold environment such as immersion in the sea or wind chill.

Signs

- Shivering in the early stages.
- Skin pale and cold.
- Temperature lower than normal.
- Irrational behaviour.
- In the later stages, unconsciousness occurs, breathing may cease and the heart may stop.

MOTORMASTER

Treatment

1 Stop further heat loss.

2 Remove to a sheltered place and take off wet clothes.

3 Replace with dry clothing, blankets or sleeping bag and wrap in a space blanket. If no dry clothing or shelter is available, cover with any material to hand such as wind-proof jackets, towels etc. Place in a horizontal position. Body heat can be transferred from another person in the sleeping bag.

4 Keep in a warm position if possible such as near a running engine or a cooker.

5 If conscious give hot sweet drinks and chocolate. Do not give alcohol or attempt to massage the skin. Raise the casualty's legs.

6 If unconscious, place in the recovery position and watch in case vomiting occurs, breathing ceases or the heart stops.

7 In case any of these things happen, be ready to take the appropriate action.

INSECT STINGS

1 Apply antihistamine cream.

2 In rare cases some people may have a severe reaction, become unconscious and stop breathing. If this happens the appropriate emergency action must be taken and medical help sought.

INTERNAL BLEEDING

This can occur through a number of reasons, such as an accident or internal disease. There is little that can be done on the boat, as medical assistance is needed as soon as possible. The VHF radio should be used to summon help.

Treatment

1 Loosen any tight clothing and lie the casualty down with head lower than the feet and to one side in case of vomiting. If possible, raise the legs, keeping them straight. This will ensure a supply of blood to vital organs.

2 Cover with a blanket, placing one beneath if necessary.

3 Check breathing and pulse rate every 10 minutes and keep a record for the doctor.

4 Reassure the casualty and observe their level of response. Encourage relaxation by slow deep breaths.

5 Be ready to take the appropriate action should breathing fail and the heart stop.

JELLYFISH STINGS

Jellyfish can inflict an extremely painful sting which swells and blisters similar to a burn. Some species can cause serious injury or death.

Treatment

Apply ammonia to the affected part.

NOSE BLEED

Treatment

1 Sit the casualty down with the body leaning forward.

2 Loosen tight clothing.

MOTORMASTER

3 Ask them to pinch the soft part of the nose and breathe through the mouth.

4 Release after 10 minutes but, if bleeding has not stopped, repeat.

5 For heavy, persistent bleeding it may be necessary to place a plug of cotton wool in the nostril.

6 Seek medical help if the bleeding does not stop.

SEASICKNESS

Seasickness is aggravated by cold, excess alcohol and lack of food.

Prevention

There are some very effective tablets available which should be started 24 hours before the passage.

Treatment

In some cases the only cure is to go ashore. It may help to occupy the casualty with something which needs concentration such as steering.

In severe cases, the casualty should lie down covered with a blanket and try to sleep.

After being seasick it is important to drink plenty of water as dehydration can quickly set in, and to eat at least small amounts. Dry bread or plain biscuits are ideal.

SEA URCHIN SPINES

Spines may become embedded quite deeply in the skin especially if the casualty has jumped on a sea urchin. At the time of the injury they cause intense pain. The wound may later become infected and need medical treatment.

Treatment

If possible remove the spines; any that have broken off will eventually be absorbed by the body.

SHOCK

Shock is caused by a reduction in the volume of blood circulating around the body or a fall in blood pressure. When this happens blood is diverted away from the extremities to vital areas. Shock accompanies most injuries and must be treated as well as the injury.

Signs

• Skin pale or grey, cold and clammy.

• Extremities cold.

• Casualty feels faint or sick.

• Pulse rapid and weak.

• Feeling of thirst.

• May become unconscious.

Treatment

1 Reassure the casualty.

2 Loosen tight clothing.

3 If conscious, lie the casualty down on their back with head to one side and raise the legs. This helps the blood to reach the brain, heart and lungs.

4 If unconscious, place in the recovery position and monitor breathing.

5 Should there be a chest injury, place in the most comfortable position.

6 Cover with a blanket.

SPRAINS

A sprain is a torn or stretched ligament or tissue around a joint.

Signs

- Pain at the joint especially when moved.
- Swelling.
- Later bruising.

Treatment

1 Immobilise in the most comfortable position and elevate if possible.

2 Apply ice cubes or a cold compress if this can be done immediately to reduce pain and swelling.

3 Pad with cotton wool and bandage.

STRAINS

A strain is the result of an overstretched muscle.

Signs

- Sudden sharp pain.
- Swelling.

Treatment

1 Rest in the most comfortable position and elevate if possible.

2 Ice cubes or a cold water compress applied for about 30 minutes may help if applied at the time of the injury.

3 Apply a bandage over cotton wool padding to reduce swelling.

SUNBURN

Treatment

1 Remove the casualty to a cool place out of the sun.

2 Sponge with cold water and apply calamine lotion.

3 Treat for heatstroke if necessary.

4 If severely burned, the casualty will need medical help.

QUESTIONS

24.1 A member of the crew has just been recovered after falling overboard. He is breathing but very cold. What action should you take?

24.2 A member of the crew has cut his wrist and it is bleeding profusely. How can you stop the bleeding and what treatment should be applied when the bleeding has stopped?

24.3 A crew member has suffered a burn on the forearm from the cooker.
a) What action should be taken immediately?
b) What further action is necessary?

24.4 What is the treatment for sunburn?

24.5 The skipper has fallen down the companionway and is suffering from severe pain in his right leg. What treatment would you apply?

MOTORMASTER

CRUISE PLANNING

Check List

Item	Done	Notes/Defects
Engine 1		
Engine 2		
Fuel		
Gas		
Water		
Props clear		
Anchor		
W/S Wipers		
Seacocks		
Dinghy		
Outboard		
VHF		
Decca		
Radar		
Compass		
Batteries		
Nav Lights		
Flares		
Extinguishers		
Lifejackets		
Liferaft		
First Aid Kit		
Customs		

CREW and GUESTS

Charts

No.	Title

Port	Entrance Waypoint	Tides		
		High Water	Hrs	Ht
		Low Water	Hrs	Ht
		High Water	Hrs	Ht
		Low Water	Hrs	Ht

Forecast — **Weather**

Time	Area	Wind	Wind later	Visibility

Actual

Time	Wind	Baro	Wave height	Visibility	Remarks

Fuel Purchased

Quantity litres	Cost	Cost per litre	Where bought

Reference Port — **Tidal Streams**

	HW	Hrs	Springs/Neaps
Time	Position	Direction	Rate

CRUISE SUMMARY

Ports visited	Elapsed Time h m		Distance travelled nautical miles		Fuel consumption litres		Average Speed knots		Remarks
	Day	Cruise	Day	Cruise	Day	Cruise	Day	Cruise	

Fig 25.1 *Example of a Cruise Planning sheet.*

PASSAGE PLANNING and DECK LOG

DATE:

FROM :

TO :

High Water	Hrs	Ht	Standard Port (Departure)			
Low Water	Hrs	Ht	High Water	Hrs	Ht	Range
			Low Water	Hrs	Ht	

High Water	Hrs	Ht	Standard Port (Destination)			
Low Water	Hrs	Ht	High Water	Hrs	Ht	Range
			Low Water	Hrs	Ht	

DOVER High Water Hrs Range

Magnetic Variation

LOG DISTANCE
START:
FINISH:

FUEL CONTENTS
START:
FINISH:

FUEL CONSUMPTION
ESTIMATED:
ACTUAL:

GROUND TRACK True	CROSS TRACK TIDE	WATER TRACK True	COMPASS ERROR	ALONG TRACK TIDE	GROUND SPEED	DISTANCE Miles	WAY POINT	WAYPOINT DESCRIPTION	COURSE TO STEER Compass	ESTIMATED ELAPSED TIME	ESTIMATED TIME OF ARRIVAL	TIME	LOG	NOTES

Cruise Speed

Fig 25.2 *Example of Passage Planning and Deck Log sheets.*

MOTORMASTER

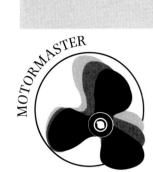

C H A P T E R   T W E N T Y   F I V E

PASSAGE PLANNING

Before embarking on any sea passage, whether it is just a trip out of the harbour or a voyage across the English Channel, it is necessary to plan things out well beforehand. The amount of pre–planning will depend on your experience; the equipment available, knowledge of the area concerned, and the length of the passage.

CHECK LISTS FOR EFFECTIVE PLANNING

A day or so before

1 Look at all charts to be used to see whether they need updating and obtain the latest Notices to Mariners to see that no corrections have been missed. A visit to the Harbour Master's office usually pays dividends as he will have details of any activities or changes within the harbour limits such as dredging or maintenance of navigational marks.

2 You will need a small scale chart initially to plan your voyage. Larger scale charts will be required for coastal passages. The largest scale charts will be required for any harbours or anchorages you might visit.

3 Check:

- Engine running
- Batteries
- Safety equipment
- Dinghy and outboard engine
- Cooking facilities
- Stores
- Bedding
- Wet weather gear

4 Start a record of the general weather pattern to build up a picture of its development.

5 Work out the starting time for the voyage, considering your local tides and daylight hours. Check the tides at the destination bearing in mind the opening times of any locks and basins. Measure the mileage, look up the tidal streams and make a rough estimate of the time to complete the passage, allowing for the boat's normal cruising speed. Fill in relevant details in the *Cruise Planning* and *Passage Planning and Deck Log* sheet (see examples in Figs 25.1 and 25.2 shown opposite).

6 Draw in the proposed track on your chart and check for any hazards on the way. If using an electronic position fixing system, mark in the waypoints. Highlight any conspicuous landmarks. For a night passage, list the characteristics together with the visibility range and bearing of all lights likely to be encountered (remembering that buoys are not generally visible at a range greater than 2 M). Establish alternative destinations in case of unforeseen circumstances.

On the day of departure

Before the passage:

- Fill up with water
- Fill fuel tanks
- Check that a spare gas bottle for the gas cooker is on board

- Get the latest weather forecast
- Fill out check list on *Cruise Planning* form
- Check that all waypoints are entered in the electronic positioning system
- Finish completing *Cruise Planning*, *Passage Planning* and *Deck Log* forms
- When departure time is confirmed, work out the DR positions (and estimated positions if you have time)
- Ensure that the crew are familiar with the location of safety equipment and emergency procedures
- Tell a responsible person ashore the details of your passage and who will be on board

After starting

1 As you clear the harbour entrance, set the log to zero and give the helmsman the course to steer. When you can establish the boat's speed, check the estimated positions for the first part of the passage. Check range and bearing of the next waypoint. Check that the course made good is compatible with your desired ground track.

2 Call the Coastguard and give details of your passage, persons on board and ETA (estimated time of arrival) to home port.

3 Fix the boat's position regularly; at least every 30 minutes if within sight of land. Compare the estimated positions and fixes to make allowance for any deviation from the desired track. Record the log reading every hour; and the barometric pressure and wind direction and speed at least every four hours. The deck log should contain sufficient navigational information so that the broad details of the passage could be recreated later.

4 If the weather conditions are deteriorating, be prepared to make for an alternative destination or to turn back.

5 When you can establish the ETA at the destination re-check any restrictions due to tidal stream or height of tide. Be prepared to anchor or pick up a mooring near the entrance. Check for local signals restricting entry to the harbour or any tidal basins.

6 Frequently, when entering an unfamiliar harbour, it is not clear where a visitor should go initially. Use of the VHF radio to call up the local marina or harbour master is ideal. If visitor's moorings or berths can be identified, they should be used. Otherwise it may be necessary to secure to a vacant buoy or pontoon so that a crew member can go ashore to seek advice on berthing. Should the owners return meanwhile, they will probably be able to give guidance on an alternative berth; but be prepared to move at short notice.

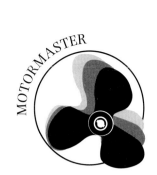

CHAPTER TWENTY-SIX

COASTAL PASSAGE PLAN: Poole to Christchurch

On 2 July we are taking a small motor cruiser from Cobbs Quay Marina in Poole to Tom Lack's Yard in Christchurch. The motor cruiser can cruise at 8 knots on her single outboard engine. Her length is 7 m and she draws 0.6 m.

PILOTAGE

Cobbs Quay Marina is situated on the west side of Hole's Bay, and is accessible on all states of the tide (top of chart extract Fig 27.12). There is a channel marked by perches (sticks in the seabed either side of the channel) through Upton Lake and down Beck Water Channel to Poole Bridge. The chart states that the marina is accessible at all states of tide but the least depth of water shown (Fig 27.12) would appear to be 01 in Upton Lake as Beck Water Channel is approached. Having passed the Town Quay at Poole turn south through the Little Channel to join the well-buoyed Middle Ship Channel which leads to the harbour entrance between North Haven and South haven Points. There is a chain ferry running across the harbour entrance which hoists a black ball forward in the direction she is travelling (see also pages 60–1).

After the prominent Haven Hotel to port there is a choice of the Swash Channel ahead or the East Looe Channel to port. The East Looe Channel is the most direct, with a possible least depth of 0.4 m close inshore. Keep parallel to the shore after the Haven Hotel until a North Cardinal beacon is passed to starboard. Head for the East Looe red buoy, leaving it close to starboard, then head 120° M to pass East Hook red buoy to starboard.

We can now follow the coast about one mile offshore (Fig 27.2) with beaches of Bournemouth to port. There are yellow buoys (marking sewer outfalls) about a mile offshore. There are no dangers to navigation as far as Hengistbury Head.

The port information for Christchurch warns of the possible danger of the Beerpan Rocks 1/2 cable (100 metres) south of the groyne leading from Hengistbury Head. If there is a strong tidal stream there could be overfalls and a choppy sea as we round Hengistbury Head but no other dangers. From Hengistbury Head we head north past five groynes (breakwaters) extending from the shore (Fig 27.1). We should see the entrance channel to Christchurch marked with spherical red and green buoys, but we should proceed to the red port hand buoy at the seaward end of the channel before turning into the entrance channel. Once in the channel, the harbour is buoyed up to Clay Pool where Tom Lack's Boatyard is just to the east of the Christchurch Quay Sailing Club (see also pages 58–9).

TIDES

Having checked the pilotage, we now need to look at the tides and tidal streams. With a shallow draught boat capable of 8 knots we will have no problems in fair weather, but we need to be aware of any possible danger areas.

Poole: From Fig 27.10, at Poole on 2 July

details of low tides are as follows:

		LW
First	0.8	0848 BST
Second	1.0	2114 BST

Looking at the tidal curve in Fig 27.13, there will be at least 1.5 m above chart datum from 1½ hours after LW to 1½ hours before LW. (1018 to 1944)

Christchurch: See Figs 7.13 and 7.14.

	LW		HW	LW	
	Time	Height	Height	Time	Height
Portsmouth GMT	0756	1.2	4.2	2021	1.5
Differences	0035–	0.7–	2.6–	0035–	0.9–
Christchurch GMT	0721	0.5	1.6	1946	0.6
Add 1 hour	0100+			0100+	
Christchurch BST	0821	0.5	1.6	2046	0.6

Range at Portsmouth: 2.8

From Fig 7.15 there will be a height of tide of at least 1.0 m except 3 hours either side of LW. So from 1121 to 1746 there will be adequate height of tide both at the entrance and throughout the harbour. There may be a fairly strong (more than 2 knots) flood tide at the entrance at LW + 2 to 3 hours (1021 to 1121).

For the departure from Poole there is no constraint from tides or tidal streams, but a departure after 1018 would allow a reasonable safety factor.

At the entrance to Christchurch the approach will be very shallow about 3 hours either side of LW, the range of the tide indicates that is about midway between neap and spring tides. There could be a flood stream (entering the harbour) 2–3 hours after LW; that is about 2 knots from 1021 to 1121.

The total distance to go is about 17 miles which could take 2½ to 3 hours. It would be preferable to enter Christchurch on the flood tide about 3 hours after LW, ie about 1121 or later. A departure from Poole sometime after 1030 would seem appropriate. It would be desirable to arrive at Christchurch at the latest 3 hours before LW, ie at 1746, which suggests a latest departure time from Poole of 1400

WEATHER

Poole Bay is open to winds from due east through south east to south. South of Hengistbury Head is exposed to south westerly winds, though the entrance to Christchurch is protected from the south west.

Any weather forecast that gives winds of more than force 3 between east and south or force 4 from the south west would indicate that the passage should not be made. Visibility should preferably be moderate (2 to 5 miles) or better.

REPORTING TO COASTGUARD

As long as the Coastguard have general details of your boat, it is not necessary for a short coastal passage to tell them directly. However, you should let a friend know your passage details, and he should be told to alert the Coastguard if you have not reported in by, say, nightfall.

MOTORMASTER

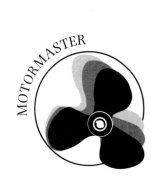

CHAPTER TWENTY-SEVEN

OFFSHORE PASSAGE MAKING: Christchurch to Cherbourg, Alderney & Poole

You are taking a Fairline 36 Turbo motor cruiser from Tom Lack's Yard in Christchurch and crossing the English Channel to France and the Channel Islands; then returning the boat to Cobb's Quay Marina in Poole. The boat's name is *Gambit*. She has a length of 12.2 m and a draught of 1.0 m. She has twin Volvo TAMD41 200 hp inboard diesel engines with twin 116 gallon fuel tanks. Her normal cruising speed in displacement mode is 8 knots and 18 knots in planing mode. On 16 July you expect to be able to get on board at 0900 and would like to motor across the Channel to Cherbourg before nightfall. The weather forecast is: wind: south to southeast force 2 to 3; weather: hazy; visibility: moderate.

PASSAGE NOTES:
Christchurch to Cherbourg, 16 July

(See Fig 27.14 for passage notes.) Study Charts 15 and 7 (Figs 27.1 and 27.2). Find Christchurch and identify the location of Tom Lack Yacht Services Boatyard at the junction of the rivers Stour and Avon. On the chart you can trace the path of the marked channel leading down the River Stour and out to sea past Mudeford Quay where it narrows between the quay and a sand spit. As you can see from the chart, the depths are shallow and entry or exit from Christchurch should be made on a rising tide. The following are extracts from the sailing directions on Chart 15:

A sandbar runs parallel to the entrance channel on the seaward side for much of its length and winds over force 4 blowing across the bar will cause seas to break into the channel and make the entrance unpleasant. Fresh onshore winds from S or SE may produce a heavy swell and entrance should not be attempted in winds of force 5 or above.

Although the channel changes greatly from year to year, there is usually at least 1 m in the entrance channel and The Run, although this depth may be reduced in prolonged N/NE winds.

Max draft for entry is about 1.1 m at HW although yachts with drafts of up to 1.5 m can enter at springs. The best entrance is made from 2 hours before HW to the 2nd HW on springs and during the stand on neaps. Entry should only be attempted on a rising tide.

Once across the bar, the channel runs in a south westerly direction with Mudeford Quay to starboard and the shingle spit to port. This part of the channel is known as The Run and it is here that the tidal streams are fiercest.

At neaps, and with little or no recent rain and/or a high barometer, the tide rises very slowly in the harbour and vessels drawing more than about 1 m are unlikely to reach the river. On a good spring tide, boats drawing up to 1.2 m can navigate the channel into the river.

Pilotage: Christchurch

With moderate visibility (5 miles or less), it is essential that the electronic navigation system is working correctly and the radar is fully operational to identify other vessels on a collision course. With the wind from the southeast there is a likelihood of some

---

Tidal heights for Christchurch
See Figs 7.13 and 7.14.

	LW Time	LW Height	HW Time	HW Height	LW Time	LW Height	Range
Portsmouth GMT	0815	0.8	1535	4.7	2041	1.3	3.9
Differences	−0035	−0.4	−0042	−2.9	−0035	−0.8	(near springs)
Christchurch	0740	0.4	1453	1.8	2006	0.5	
Add 1 hour	0100		0100		0100		
Christchurch BST	0840	0.4	1553	1.8	2106	0.5	

The height of tide required to clear the bar in the entrance channel (charted depth 0_1) will be: $1.0 + 0.5 - 0.1 = 1.4$ m (draught + safe clearance − charted depth). Fill in the tidal curve diagram, Fig 7.15. Earliest time to cross the bar is LW + 3 hrs or 1140. The latest time to cross the bar is LW − 3 hrs or 1806.

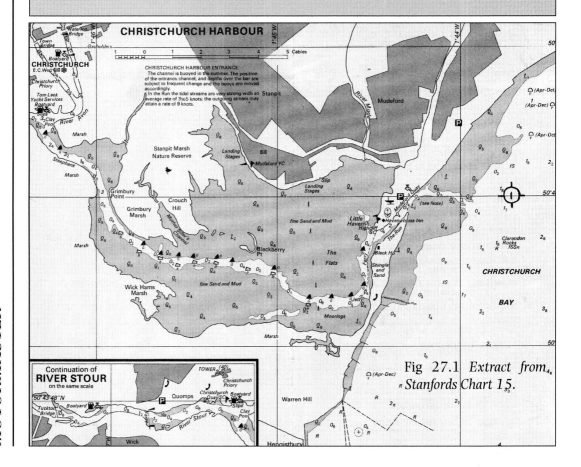

Fig 27.1 *Extract from Stanfords Chart 15.*

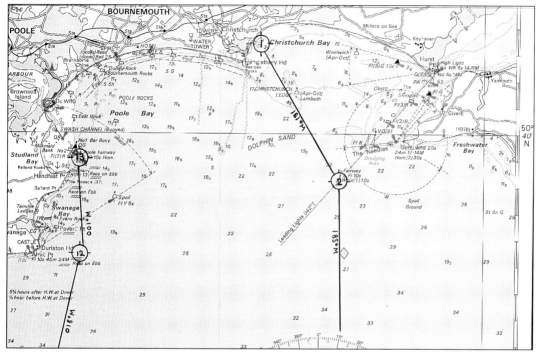

Fig 27.2 *Extract from Stanfords Chart 7 showing Poole Bay.*

swell in the shallow waters in the harbour entrance and in Christchurch Bay beyond. Extending from Hengistbury Head is Christchurch Ledge which may cause a disturbed sea but no danger in a force 3 wind as long as Beerpan Rocks are left well clear. We will need some clearing bearings or clearing transits for this.

Tidal streams

In 'The Run' at the entrance to Christ- church Harbour, at spring tides the tidal stream can flood at a rate of 3 knots between LW+2 and LW+3: that is from 1040 to 1140. If departure from the Boatyard is timed for 1130, then the harbour entrance will be reached just after 1145 which will avoid the full strength of the tidal stream and will have sufficient height of tide to clear the bar.

Dover and Cherbourg HW and LW times. (From Figs 27.3 and 27.4)						
	HW		**LW**		**HW**	
	Time	Height	Time	Height	Time	Height
Cherbourg BST	1244	5.7	1930	1.5		
Dover GMT	0237	6.3			1450	6.4
Dover BST	0337	6.3			1550	6.4
	Range at Dover: (6.4 − 0.9) = 5.5 (near springs)					

MOTORMASTER

CHERBOURG

HIGH & LOW WATER

JULY

	Time	m		Time	m
1 W	0621 1156 1840	1.9 5.3 2.0	**16** TH	0021 0708 1244 1930	6.2 1.3 5.7 1.5
2 TH	0015 0700 1234 1920	5.4 2.0 5.2 2.1	**17** F	0107 0754 1331 2019	5.9 1.6 5.5 1.8
3 F	0055 0741 1318 2004	5.3 2.1 5.1 2.2	**18** SA	0156 0846 1422 2115	5.5 1.9 5.2 2.1
4 SA	0141 0830 1406 2058	5.2 2.2 5.1 2.3	**19** SU	0251 0946 1524 2221	5.3 2.2 5.0 2.4
5 SU	0234 0927 1503 2158	5.2 2.3 5.0 2.3	**20** M	0359 1056 1637 2332	5.0 2.5 4.9 2.5
6 M	0336 1032 1609 2304	5.2 2.3 5.1 2.2	**21** TU	0513 1207 1749	4.9 2.5 5.0

TIME ZONE – 0100 SUBTRACT 1 HOUR FOR GMT

Fig 27.3 *Extract from tide tables for Cherbourg.*

Tidal streams: *Christchurch Bay* (see Fig 27.5)
Eastbound starts HW Dover+6 = 0937
  (max rate at HW–4: 2.1 knots)
Westbound starts HW Dover = 1550
  (max rate at HW+2: 2.3 knots)

Mid-Channel
Eastbound starts HW Dover+6 = 0937/ 2150
  (max rate at HW–2: 2.5 knots)
Westbound starts HW Dover = 1550
  (max rate HW+2: 3 knots)

Off Cherbourg
Eastbound starts HW Dover+6 = 2150
  (max rate at HW–3: 5 knots)
Westbound starts HW Dover = 1550
  (max rate HW+4: 6 knots)

Fig 27.4 *Extract from Dover tide tables.*

Lat. 51°07′N.   Long. 1°19′E.

DOVER

HIGH & LOW WATER

	MAY			MAY			JUNE			JUNE			JULY			JULY			AUGUST			AUGUST	
	Time	m		Time	m		Time	m		Time	m		Time	m		Time	m		Time	m		Time	m
1 F	0036 0757 1300 2006	6.4 0.9 6.2 1.1	**16** Sa	0017 0745 1248 2008	6.4 0.8 6.1 0.9	**1** M	0120 0840 1348 2101	5.8 1.4 5.9 1.5	**16** Tu	0208 0934 1426 2159	6.2 1.0 6.3 0.9	**1** W	0138 0857 1405 2121	5.9 1.5 6.1 1.4	**16** Th	0237 1013 1450 2235	6.3 1.0 6.4 0.9	**1** Sa	0223 0934 1442 2202	5.9 1.6 6.1 1.5	**16** Su	0335 1040 1552 2313	5.9 1.7 6.0 1.7
2 Sa	0107 0827 1331 2042	6.2 1.1 6.0 1.3	**17** Su	0109 0833 1341 2057	6.3 0.9 6.2 1.0	**2** Tu	0157 0915 1427 2141	5.6 1.6 5.8 1.7	**17** W	0300 1028 1517 2254	6.1 1.2 6.1 1.1	**2** Th	0219 0929 1444 2159	5.7 1.6 6.0 1.5	**17** F	0324 1052 1539 2319	6.1 1.3 6.2 1.2	**2** Su	0304 1011 1524 2244	5.7 1.8 5.9 1.7	**17** M	0431 1122 1654	5.5 2.1 5.6
3 Su	0137 0901 1405 2118	6.2 1.4 5.8 1.6	**18** M	0206 0925 1434 2152	6.0 1.2 6.0 1.2	**3** W	0242 0955 1515 2224	5.4 1.8 5.6 1.8	**18** Th	0356 1123 1612 2353	5.9 1.4 5.9 1.2	**3** F	0305 1006 1531 2240	5.6 1.8 5.8 1.7	**18** Sa	0416 1134 1633	5.9 1.6 6.0	**3** M	0356 1055 1620 2337	5.5 2.0 5.7 1.9	**18** Tu	0005 0546 1225 1819	2.2 5.2 2.4 5.2
4 M	0212 0938 1447 2159	5.5 1.7 5.5 1.9	**19** Tu	0307 1026 1531 2257	5.8 1.5 5.8 1.4	**4** Th	0342 1041 1614 2318	5.2 2.0 5.5 1.9	**19** F	0459 1221 1716	5.7 1.5 5.8	**4** Sa	0400 1049 1624 2329	5.5 1.9 5.7 1.7	**19** Su	0008 0516 1224 1737	1.5 5.6 1.9 5.7	**4** Tu	0459 1158 1727	5.4 2.2 5.5	**19** W	0126 0710 1359 1944	2.4 5.2 2.4 5.2
5 Tu	0301 1020 1545 2249	5.2 2.1 5.2 2.1	**20** W	0414 1136 1637	5.6 1.6 5.6	**5** F	0452 1136 1719	5.1 2.1 5.4	**20** Sa	0055 0608 1323 1824	1.4 5.6 1.7 5.8	**5** Su	0458 1143 1720	5.4 2.1 5.7	**20** M	0107 0627 1328 1850	1.8 5.4 2.1 5.6	**5** W	0046 0612 1319 1845	2.0 5.3 2.2 5.4	**20** Th	0254 0820 1524 2051	2.4 5.3 2.2 5.4
6 W	0419 1115 1701 2354	4.9 2.3 5.1 2.2	**21** Th	0010 0539 1250 1800	1.5 5.5 1.6 5.5	**6** Sa	0021 0557 1243 1819	1.9 5.2 2.1 5.5	**21** Su	0201 0712 1426 1928	1.5 5.6 1.9 5.8	**6** M	0028 0557 1248 1819	1.8 5.4 2.1 5.7	**21** Tu	0219 0737 1443 2001	2.0 5.4 2.1 5.6	**6** Th	0206 0740 1449 2009	2.0 5.4 2.0 5.6	**21** F	0357 0917 1620 2145	2.1 5.6 1.9 5.6
7 Th	0550 1227 1817	4.8 2.4 5.1	**22** F	0127 0659 1404 1914	1.4 5.6 1.5 5.7	**7** Su	0127 0653 1349 1914	1.8 5.4 2.0 5.7	**22** M	0305 0809 1525 2026	1.5 5.7 1.7 5.9	**7** Tu	0133 0657 1359 1920	1.8 5.5 2.1 5.7	**22** W	0327 0839 1546 2101	2.0 5.6 2.0 5.6	**7** F	0332 0903 1614 2124	1.7 5.7 1.6 5.9	**22** Sa	0447 1000 1705 2224	1.8 5.9 1.5 5.8

WHEN TO ENTER — The best time is between –0200 and +0100 (Dover).
WHEN TO LEAVE — All times suitable, but caution required when meeting stream off ent.
RATE AND SET — The stream in the entrance and harbour vary considerably. E. going stream begins –0210 (Dover). Sets 068°, 4 knots (Springs), 2½ knots (Neaps). W. going stream begins +0430 (Dover). Sets 224°. 2½ knots (Springs), 1½ knots (Neaps).

MOTORMASTER

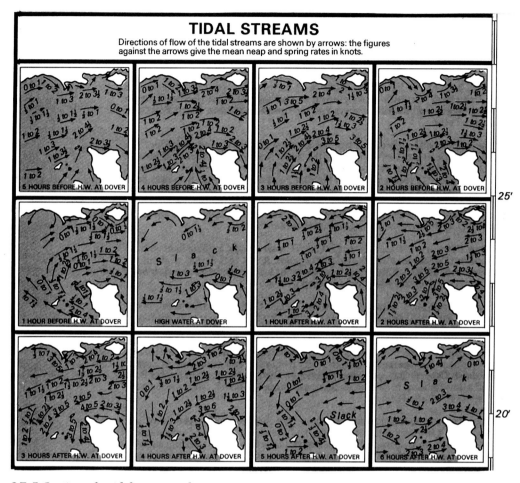

Fig 27.5 *Section of a tidal stream atlas.*

Passage: Tom Lack Yacht Services Boatyard, Christchurch, to Cherbourg Yacht Harbour

See Stanfords Chart 15 (Fig 27.1)

Start not before 1130.

Motor slowly (not more than 6 knots) out of the harbour until well clear of entrance.

See Stanfords Chart 7 (Fig 27.2)

Christchurch entrance to Needles Fairway buoy

Course 155°T, distance 6 miles

Variation is 6°W: add to true course to obtain magnetic (or compass) course = 161° M

At 18 knots, time taken = 20 mins

See Stanfords Chart 7 (Fig 27.6)

Needles Fairway buoy to Cherbourg outer breakwater (west entrance)

Course 179°T (185° M), distance 58 miles

At 18 knots, time taken = 3 hours 14 mins

From Christchurch entrance, time taken to reach Cherbourg west entrance is just over 3 hours 30 minutes.

MOTORMASTER

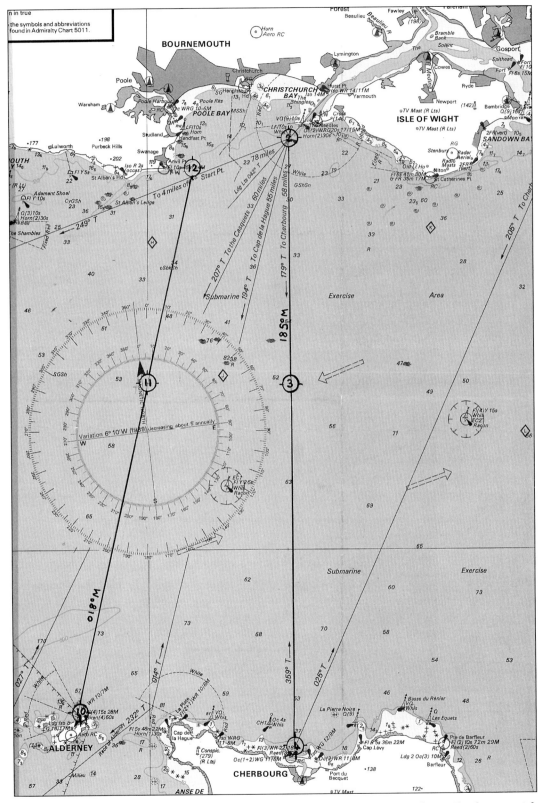

Fig 27.6 *Part of Stanfords Chart 7 showing passage from Christchurch to Cherbourg with waypoints.*

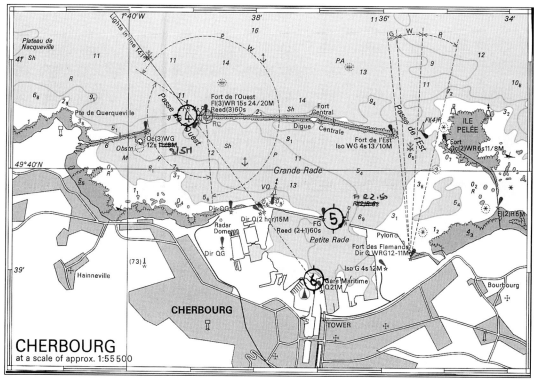

Fig 27.7 Cherbourg harbour plan.

Note that, based on a departure time of 1200 from Christchurch entrance, there is likely to be an eastbound set of the tidal stream of about 2 knots, gradually slackening off from mid-Channel. Watch out for eastgoing and westgoing shipping south of the mid-Channel waypoint. EC1 buoy in mid-Channel will be passed about 6 miles to starboard about 30 minutes after the mid-Channel waypoint; but it is unlikely to be visible.

Cherbourg Harbour

Approaches to Cherbourg: see Stanfords Chart 7 (Fig 27.6) and harbour plan (Fig 27.7). Cherbourg peninsula has high

ground at its northwest and northeast corners, but the port and town of Cherbourg is fairly low-lying. The first sighting of land, therefore, could well be the high ground on the northwest corner of the peninsula in the area of the chimney (279 m above sea level) shown on Chart 7. The line of the outer breakwater, with the fort at its western end, is easy to identify. The CH1 buoy 3 miles northwest of the entrance, may be sighted at a distance about 2 miles to starboard.

The voyage is continued two days later. The weather forecast is for westerly winds, force 3-4, with good visibility.

MOTORMASTER

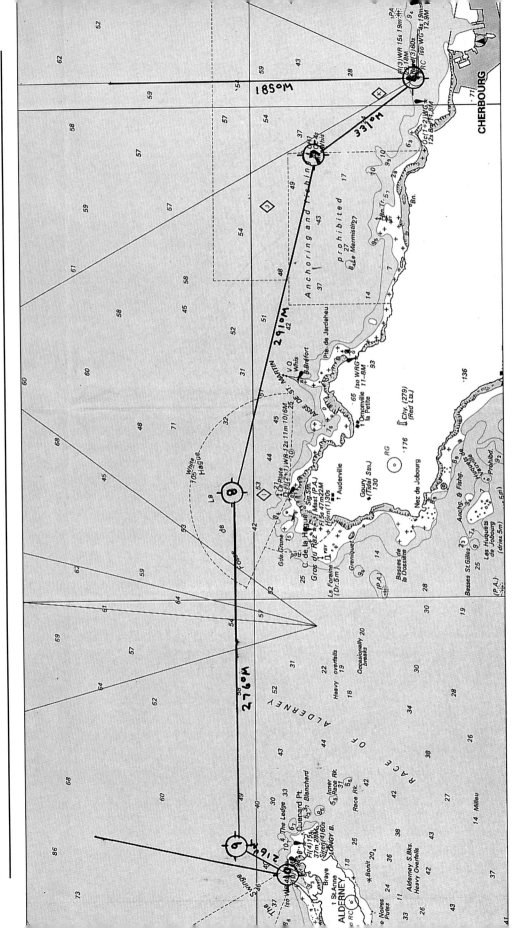

Fig 27.8 *Passage from Cherbourg to Alderney marked on Stanfords Chart 7.*

PASSAGE NOTES: CHERBOURG TO ALDERNEY, 18 JULY
Tides See Figs 27.3, 27.4, 27.9 and 27.11

HW Dover	GMT	0416	5.9	1633	6.0	Range: (5.9−1.6) = 4.3
	BST	0516	5.9	1733	6.0	between spring and neap tides
HW Cherbourg BST	0156		5.5	1422	5.2	
LW Cherbourg BST	0846		1.9			

Tide Tables: St Helier

	HW		LW		HW	
St Helier GMT	1143	8.8	1824	3.5	0010	8.7
Tidal difference for Alderney	+0045	−3.7	+0050	−1.3	+0045	−3.7
Alderney GMT	1228	5.1	1914	2.2	0055	5.0
(Braye Harbour) BST	1328	5.1	2014	2.2	0155	5.0

Tidal streams:
Off Cherbourg

Westbound starts HW Dover = 1733
   (max rate at HW+4: 4.5 knots)

Off Alderney
Southwest bound starts HW Dover = 1733
Northeast bound starts HW Dover+6 = 2333

(Note: consult larger scale tidal stream atlas for greater detail.)

Passage: Cherbourg Yacht Harbour to Braye Harbour, Alderney

Because of the possibility of rough seas between Cherbourg and Alderney (particularly if the wind is blowing against the tidal stream), you decide to make the passage at displacement speed (8 knots).

As the westbound tidal stream starts at 1733 (in practice there is a westbound tidal stream inshore about 1 hour earlier), the planned time for leaving Cherbourg yacht harbour is 1700 in order to pass the outer breakwater at 1730.

See Stanfords Chart 7 (Fig 27.8)
   Cherbourg breakwater to CH1 buoy
   Course 325°T (331°M), distance 3 miles
   At 8 knots, time taken = 23 mins

MOTORMASTER

CH1 buoy to 1 mile north of La Platte beacon tower
  Course 285°T (291°M), distance 9 miles
  At 8 knots, time taken = 1 hour 8 mins
1 mile north of La Platte beacon tower to 2 miles north of Quenard Point lighthouse
  270°T (276°M), distance 9 miles
  At 8 knots, time taken = 1 hour 8 mins
2 miles north of Quenard Point lighthouse to Braye harbour
  210°T (216°M), distance 2 miles
  At 8 knots, time taken = 15 mins

Estimated passage time from Cherbourg breakwater to Braye harbour at 8 knots is just under 3 hours. A favourable tidal stream averaging 2.5 knots could reduce the passage time by 40 minutes.

Approaches to Alderney

The prominent white lighthouse at Quenard Point is easily visible. There can be some rough seas and strong tidal streams around Alderney, so steering a steady course may not be easy. Keeping about 2 miles offshore, proceed around the northeast corner of Alderney until the entrance to Braye harbour (inside the breakwater) is clearly visible. There are leading marks for the entrance which can be identified from a large scale chart of the harbour plan. Be aware that the breakwater extends underwater for 0.3 miles.

The voyage is continued to Poole two days later. The weather is fine with a light breeze from the southwest.

PASSAGE NOTES: ALDERNEY TO POOLE, 20 JULY
Tides See Figs 27.4, 27.9, 27.10 and 27.11

HW Dover GMT	0627	5.4	1850	5.6	Range (5.4−2.1) = 3.3
BST	0727	5.4	1950	5.6	neap tides
LW Poole GMT	1211	1.1	0047	1.1	
BST	1311	1.1	0147	1.1	

Tidal streams: Off north coast of Alderney
Eastbound starts HW Dover+5 = 1227
Westbound starts HW Dover = 0727

Mid-Channel
Eastbound starts HW Dover+6 = 1327
  (max rate at HW −3: 1 knot)
Westbound starts HW Dover = 0727/1950
  (max rate at HW+2: 2 knots)

Approaches to Poole
Southwest bound starts HW Dover = 1950
  (max rate at HW+2: 1.3 knots)
Northeast bound starts HW Dover+6 = 1327
  (max rate at HW −4: 1.3 knots)

ST. HELIER JERSEY

HIGH & LOW WATER

JULY

	Time	m		Time	m
1	0343	2·7	**16**	0434	1·6
	0927	9·2		1010	10·1
W	1552	3·0	Th	1652	2·4
	2136	9·4		2230	10·0
2	0414	2·9	**17**	0516	2·3
	1000	9·0		1054	9·4
Th	1626	3·3	F	1734	3·0
	2213	9·2		2316	9·4
3	0448	3·2	**18**	0601	3·0
	1038	8·8		1143	8·8
F	1704	3·5	Sa	1824	3·5
	2255	8·9			
4	0526	3·5	**19**	0010	8·7
	1126	8·6		0655	3·6
Sa	1751	3·8	Su	1241	8·3
	2347	8·6		1924	3·9
5	0618	3·7	**20**	0114	8·3
	1224	8·4		0759	3·9
Su	1853	3·9	M	1351	8·1
				2033	4·0
6	0049	8·5	**21**	0230	8·1
	0726	3·8		0905	4·0
M	1333	8·5	Tu	1503	8·2
	2005	3·7		2139	3·8

Fig 27.9 *Extract from St Helier tide tables.*

POOLE

LOW WATER

JULY

	TIME	M		TIME	M
1	0710	1.9	**16**	0808	2.1
		0.7			0.5
W	1932	2.0	TH	2035	2.2
		1.0			0.9
2	0748	1.9	**17**	0900	2.1
		0.8			0.7
TH	2014	2.0	F	2129	2.1
		1.0			0.9
3	0831	1.8	**18**	0957	1.9
		0.9			0.9
F	2101	1.9	SA	2232	2.0
		1.1			1.1
4	0921	1.8	**19**	1104	1.8
		0.9			1.9
SA	2156	1.9	SU	2339	1.9
		1.1			1.1
5	1021	1.8	**20**	1211	1.8
		1.0			1.1
SU	2300	1.9	M		1.9
		1.1			
6	1129	1.8	**21**	0047	1.1
		1.1			1.8
M		1.9	TU	1317	1.2
					1.9

GMT ADD 1 HOUR MARCH 29
— OCTOBER 25 FOR B.S.T.

Fig 27.10 *Extract from a tide table for Poole.*

TIDAL DIFFERENCES ON ST. HELIER

PLACE	TIME DIFFERENCES				HEIGHT DIFFERENCES (Metres)			
	High Water		Low Water		MHWS	MHWN	MLWN	MLWS
ST. HELIER .... CHANNEL ISLANDS	0300 and 1500	0900 and 2100	0200 and 1400	0900 and 2100	11.1	8.1	4.1	1.3
Alderney Braye	+0050	+0040	+0025	+0105	−4.8	−3.4	−1.5	−0.5

Fig 27.11 *Table of tidal differences for St Helier.*

Passage: Alderney, Braye Harbour, to Poole, Cobbs Quay Marina

No constraints on departure or arrival times. With neap tides (Fig 27.9), tidal streams are insignificant. It is decided to leave Braye harbour at 1400.

See Stanfords Chart 7 (Fig 27.6)
Alderney (Braye harbour) to 2 miles east of Anvil Point lighthouse
Course 012°T (018°M), distance 54 miles
At 18 knots, time taken = 3 hours

MOTORMASTER

MOTORMASTER

PARKSTONE BAY

Lower Hamworthy

Hamworthy Park

CHIMNEYS (99) (99) Power Station

St James Church TOWER FS

Town Quay

Westons Pt
Parkstone YC
Lilliput SC
Blue Lagoon
Poole Harbour YC

Spherical Tank (20)

Poole Br (opening – see Note)
Wharves

Poole YC
Continental Freight Quay
New Channel
Ferry Terminal
Little Channel
Wills Cut

Dries Oyster Bank
Breakwater Moorings
Baiter Pt

Oyster Beds (see note)

No 55 Stakes
No 39
Parkstone YC
No 37
No 35
Salterns Marina
Lilliput Yacht Sta
Outfalls

Middle Ship Channel

Parkstone Shoal
Salterns Middle Ground

MIDDLE SHIP CHANNEL

No 54

NORTH CHANNEL

Middle Mud

WYCH CHANNEL

Survey Bn

Maryland
Jetty (ruins)
Pier (ruins)

BROWNSEA ISLAND (National Trust)

Fire Tr (41)
Mon (24)

Lincoln Cliff
Shard Pt

Blood Alley Lake

Whiteground Lake

Aunt Betty
Basket Boom
Bullpit
North Haven
Jack Jones
Royal Motor YC
Brownsea Road
Brownsea Castle (24)
N Haven Pt
Sandbanks
HAVEN HOTEL
S Haven Pt
Shell Bay
No 12A

Ramshorn Lake

Oyster Beds (see note)

Marsh

Furzey I
Marsh

Landing stage (ruin)
Foul
Oyster Beds (see note)

Green I

Pier (ruins)

Goathorn Pt
Stanley Green

Stone Island Lake
Gravel Pt
Houseboat Moorings
Jerry's Pt
Bramble Bush Bay

The Little Sea

Milkmaid Bank

Sand Dunes

Survey Bn

Beach Huts

HOLES BAY

Pergins I
Mud
Sterte

Marsh

Creekmore Lake
Upton Lake
Moorings
Obstn

Cobbs Quay Marina
Pylons

Back Water Channel
Wks (0.4)

Pile Moorings
Marina

Power

CHIMNEYS (99) (99) Power Station

Hamworthy

Lower Hamworthy

St James Church TOWER FS
Town Quay

Poole Br (opening)

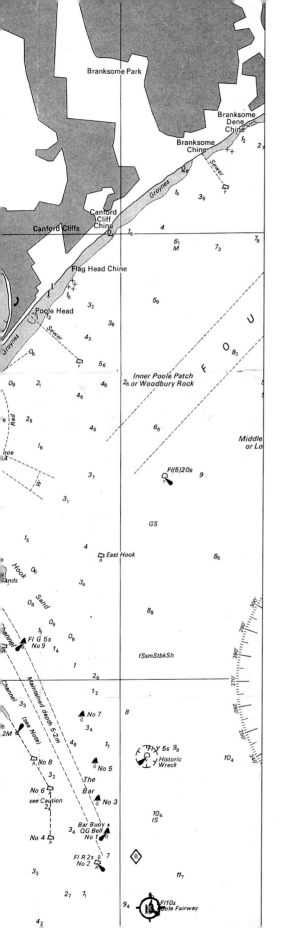

Fig 27.12 *Extract from Stanfords Chart 15 showing the approaches to Poole Harbour. Insert: Holes Bay showing Cobbs Quay Marina.*

Watch out for shipping prior to mid–Channel waypoint)
2 miles east of Anvil Point lighthouse to Poole Fairway buoy
Course 355°T (001°M), distance 4 miles
At 18 knots, time taken = 15 mins
Estimated time of Arrival (ETA) at Poole Fairway buoy: 1715

Approaches to Poole and Poole Harbour

See Figs 27.12 (Chart 15). From Poole Fairway buoy, follow the channel past Haven Point (watch out for the chain ferry) and Brownsea Island to Poole town. There may be a delay passing Poole bridge. Beyond Back Water channel the charted depth in the approaches to Cobbs Quay Marina is shown as low as 0_1 m, so you will need to calculate the actual water depth carefully (see diagram on page 230).

From the Poole tidal curve diagram (Fig 27.13) we can see that on mean neaps there is up to 1.6 m height of tide anything up to 5 hours after HW and 1½ hours before HW. As you expect to arrive at Poole at about 1715, you should find plenty of water.

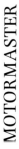

MOTORMASTER

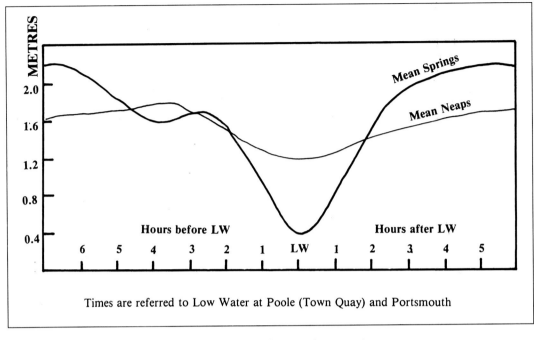

Fig 27.13 *Graph showing the rise and fall of tide at Poole Town Quay.*

IS THERE ENOUGH WATER?

If you need to motor down a shallow channel you will need to check that there is sufficient water. Knowing that your draught is 1 m and adding on 0.5 m for clearance; then deduct the lowest charted depth which in this example is 0_1:

$1 m + 0.5 m - 0.1 = 1.4$

So you now know that you will need at least 1.4 metres tidal

height to pass safely down the channel

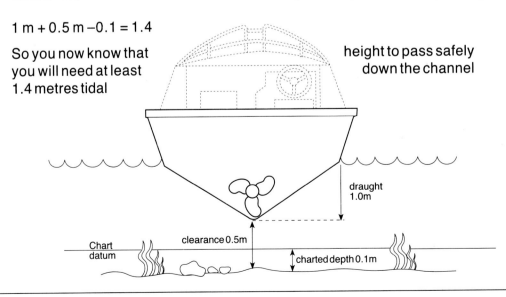

WAYPOINTS LIST

Route: Christchurch to Cherbourg

WP No	Description	Latitude	Longitude	Next WP Course °M	Dist Miles	Time elapsed	Time taken (at 18 knots)
1	Christchurch entrance	50°43.5N	1°43.7W	161	6	20 mins	
2	Needles Fairway buoy	50°38.2N	1°38.9W	185	23	1 hr 17 mins	20 mins
3	Mid-Channel	50°15.0N	1°39.0W	185	35	1 hr 57 mins	1 hr 37 mins
4	Cherbourg W b'water	49°40.5N	1°39.0W	127	1.7	–	3 hr 34 mins
5	Inner hbr b'water	49°39.6N	1°36.7W	204	0.6	–	–
6	Yacht hbr	49°39.0N	1°37.0W	–	–	–	–

Route: Cherbourg to Alderney

WP No	Description	Latitude	Longitude	Next WP Course °M	Dist Miles	Time elapsed	Time taken (at 8 knots)
4	Cherbourg W b'water	49°40.5N	1°39.0W	331	3	23 mins	–
7	CH1 buoy	49°43.3N	1°42.1W	291	9	1 hr 8 mins	23 mins
8	1M N of La Platte Beacon	49°45.0N	1°55.7W	276	9	1 hr 8 mins	1 hr 31 mins
9	2M N of Quenard Pt	49°45.8N	2°09.8W	216	2	15 mins	2 hr 39 mins
10	Braye hbr	49°44.1N	2°11.1W	–	–	–	2 hr 54 mins

Route: Alderney to Poole

WP No	Description	Latitude	Longitude	Next WP Course °M	Dist Miles	Time elapsed	Time taken (at 18 knots)
10	Braye hbr	49°44.1N	2°11.1W	018	31	1 hr 43 mins	–
11	Mid-Channel	50°15.0N	2°02.0W	018	23	1 hr 7 mins	1 hr 43 mins
12	2M E of Anvil Pt	50°35.6N	1°54.3W	001	4	13 mins	3 hrs
13	Poole Fairway buoy	50°39.0N	1°54.8W	Var	2	–	3 hr 13 mins
14	Poole hbr entrance	50°40.8N	1°56.7W	–	–	–	–

MOTORMASTER

PASSAGE PLANNING and DECK LOG

DATE: 16 JULY

FROM: CHRISTCHURCH   TO: CHERBOURG

High Water 1553 Hrs 1.8 Ht	Standard Port (Departure) PORTSMOUTH	High Water 1244 Hrs 5.7 Ht	Standard Port (Destination)
Low Water 0840 Hrs 0.4 Ht	High Water 1635 Hrs 4.7 Ht Range	Low Water 1930 Hrs 1.5 Ht	High Water Hrs Ht Range
	Low Water 0815 Hrs 0.8 Ht 3.9		Low Water Hrs Ht

DOVER High Water 1550 Hrs	LOG DISTANCE	FUEL CONTENTS	FUEL CONSUMPTION
Range 5.5	START: 0.0	START: 1000	ESTIMATED: 247
Magnetic Variation 6°W	FINISH: 67.8	FINISH: 753	ACTUAL:

GROUND TRACK True	CROSS TRACK TIDE	WATER TRACK True	COMPASS ERROR	ALONG TRACK TIDE	GROUND SPEED	DISTANCE Miles	WAY POINT	WAYPOINT DESCRIPTION	COURSE TO STEER Compass	ESTIMATED ELAPSED TIME	ESTIMATED TIME OF ARRIVAL	TIME	LOG	NOTES
							0	TOM LACKS YARD				1130	0.0	
Van	—	Van	6°W	NIL	6	1.5	1	CHRISTCHURCH ENTRANCE	VAR	15	1145			
155	—	155			18	6	2	NEEDLES FAIRWAY	161	20	1205			
179	2.5↑	181			18	23	3	MID CHANNEL	187	1 17	1322			
179	1.5↑	180			18	35	4	CHERBOURG B'WATER	186	1 57	1519			
121	—	121			8	1.7	5	INNER B'WATER	127	13	1532			
198	—	198	↓	↓	8	0.6	6	YACHT HARBOUR	204	5	1537			
						67.8				4 07			Cruise Speed 18	

Diversion Ports

CRUISE PLANNING

Check List		
Item	Done	Notes/Defects
Engine 1		
Engine 2		
Fuel		
Gas		
Water		
Props clear		
Anchor		
W/S Wipers		
Seacocks		
Dinghy		
Outboard		
VHF		
Decca		
Radar		
Compass		
Batteries		
Nav Lights		
Flares		
Extinguishers		
Lifejackets		
Liferaft		
First Aid Kit		
Customs		

CREW and GUESTS

Port	Entrance Waypoint	Tides		
		High Water	Hrs	Ht
		Low Water	Hrs	Ht
		High Water	Hrs	Ht
		Low Water	Hrs	Ht

Forecast			Weather		
Time	Area		Wind	Wind later	Visibility
0555	WIGHT, PORTLAND, PLYMOUTH		S2	SE3	MOD

Actual					
Time	Wind	Baro	Wave height	Visibility	Remarks

Charts

No.	Title
15	POOLE HARBOUR & APPROACHES
7	ENGLISH CHANNEL CENTRAL SECTION

Fuel Purchased				Reference Port	Tidal Streams		
Quantity litres	Cost	Cost per litre	Where bought	DOVER	HW 1550 Hrs (Springs) Neaps		
				Time	Position	Direction	Rate
				1150	CHRISTCHURCH BAY	098°	2.1
				1350	MID CHANNEL	090°	2.5
				1250	OFF CHERBOURG	090°	5.0

CRUISE SUMMARY

Ports visited	Elapsed Time h m		Distance travelled nautical miles		Fuel consumption litres		Average Speed knots		Remarks
	Day	Cruise	Day	Cruise	Day	Cruise	Day	Cruise	
CHRISTCHURCH, CHERBOURG	4.07	4.07	67.8	67.8	247	247	16.5	16.5	

MOTORMASTER

CUSTOMS AND EXCISE

UNITED KINGDOM

Full details of United Kingdom Customs procedures and allowances are published in Notice 8B entitled *Sailing your pleasure craft to and from the United Kingdom* obtainable from HM Customs and Excise.

Between European Union countries for nationals of these countries there are no Customs formalities. However, if any crew member is not a national of an EU country, or if it is intended to import any restricted goods, birds or animals, the local Customs should be contacted.

Before visiting any non-EU country, including the Channel Islands, Form C1331 sections (i) and (ii) must be completed with the top copy being posted at a Customs check point before departure. On return, section (iii) should be completed before the 12 mile limit is reached. At the 12 mile limit, international code flag Q 'Quebec' is flown (suitably illuminated after dark). On reaching the home destination, the local Customs office must be contacted.

FOREIGN CUSTOMS

Generally the formalities between EU countries are similar to the UK but there are variations which should be checked before entry, especially as they change periodically. Some countries require an International Certificate of Competence. It is customary but not essential in some countries to fly international code flag 'Quebec' until cleared by Customs.

If the boat is registered, the registration papers (including the Bill of Sale) should be carried when going foreign. It is a wise precaution to obtain a certificate or appropriate form to verify that Value Added Tax has been paid on your boat. For information on cruising abroad, obtain a copy of the publication *Planning a Foreign Cruise* published by the Cruising Association and Royal Yachting Association.

Opposite above: Fig 27.14 *An example of a Passage Planning and Deck Log sheet for a passage from Christchurch to Cherbourg.*

Opposite below: Fig.27.15 *An example of a Cruise Planning sheet for a passage from Christchurch to Cherbourg. Note: allowance is made for cross-tide in mid Channel.*

ANSWERS TO QUESTIONS

Chapter 3

3.1 Engine horsepower/displacement in tons

$$= \frac{2 \times 320}{16} = 40$$

From Fig 3.1, Maximum boat speed = 5.8 $\sqrt{49}$ = **40.6 knots**

3.2 Engine horsepower/Displacement in tons = $\frac{76}{34}$ = 2.2

From Fig 3.1, Maximum boat speed = 1.5 $\sqrt{60}$ = **11.6 knots**

3.3 Fig A3.3 shows a series of curves for different boat speeds. At the most economical cruising speed (on the plane) of around 24 knots, the operating range on a full load of fuel would be about 125 miles or about 5 hours. At full power the range is reduced to 80 miles or just over 2 hours.

Chapter 4

4.1 A compass is affected by the earth's magnetic field, which causes variation, and the boat's magnetic field, which causes deviation.

4.2 **5° 35′W**

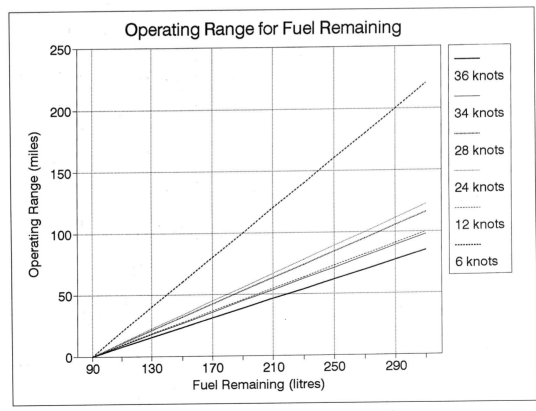

Fig A 3.3

4.3   a) **224°M**, **143°M**, **009°M**
      b) **352°T**, **185°T**, **012°T**

4.4   a) **001°C, 004°C, 158°C**
      b) **231°M, 066°M, 289°M**

4.5   From Fig 4.4, deviation for a course of 060°C is 4°E. Variation is 6°W.
      Compass Error = 6°W − 3°E = 3°W
      a) The true bearings are:
      Tower   **088°T**
      Church   **164°T**
      Monument   **327°T**
      b) **3°W**

4.6   The sensor should be well away (1 m) from ferrous metal or objects with strong magnetic fields particularly those which move as the boat pitches or rolls.

Chapter 5

5.1   Chart No 15 is a larger scale chart than chart No 12 and therefore includes more detail.

5.2   The English Channel.

5.3   Longitude scale

5.4   By referring to the latitude and longitude scales.

5.5   **1** The equator appears as a straight line.
      2 Parallels of latitude are straight lines equidistant from the Equator.
      3 Meridians of longitude are straight lines crossing the parallels at right angles.
      4 Any track on a mercator projection chart crosses all meridians at the same angle.

5.6   There is too much distortion.

5.7   The Greenwich meridian which passes through London.

5.8   *Symbols and Abbreviations used on Admiralty Charts (5011)* or US *Nautical Chart Symbols and Abbreviations, Chart No 1.*

5.9   Commercially published charts are corrected by using information obtained from the publisher. Other charts are corrected by reference to the appropriate *Notices to Mariners.*

5.10 **50° 38′.5**

Chapter 6

6.1   On a Mercator projection chart, minutes of latitude are spaced progressively further apart as latitude increases.

6.2   Anvil Point light.

6.3   **50° 36′.5N   1° 57′.0W**

6.4   **50° 36′.0N   1° 55′.0W**

6.5   a)   **014°T**
      b)   **1.4M**
      c)   Tidal race on ebb

6.6   a)   **067°T**
      b)   **0.7M**
      c)   **5min**

6.7   It is a symbol for a tidal diamond.

6.8   a)   **216°T**
      b)   **0.5M**

Chapter 7

7.1   The lowest level to which the tide is expected to fall due to astronomical conditions.

7.2   Yes. Due to abnormal weather conditions such as high barometric pressure or a strong wind blowing out of an estuary over a period of several days.

7.3   a) The depth of water between chart datum and the seabed, Fig 7.4.

MOTORMASTER

b) By figures in metres and decimetres, eg 7₃

7.4   Mean High Water Springs.

7.5   At spring tides just after the full or new moon.

7.6   From a tide table, Fig 7.6.

7.7   **3.8 metres**

7.8   **4.2 metres**

	HW		LW	Range
Dover GMT	1517	6.1	1.1	5.0 (0.3
	+0100			from
BST	1617			springs)

Interval: HW + 3hrs 03 mins

7.9   **1228 BST**

	HW		LW	Range
Dover GMT	1348	5.9	1.4	4.4 (0.5
Difference	+0020	−1.6	−0.6	from
Ramsgate				springs)
GMT	1408	4.3	0.8	
	+0100			
BST	1508			

Interval: HW −2hrs 40mins

7.10   **1.3 metres**

	HW	LW		Range
Portsmouth				
GMT	4.0	0738	1.3	1.7 (neaps)
Difference	−1.4	−0027	−0.2	
Yarmouth GMT	2.6	0711	1.1	
		+0100		
BST		0811		

Interval: LW + 2hrs 04mins

7.11   **276°T 2.6kn**

7.12   There is very little tidal stream in the bay and the boats are wind rode (lying head to wind).

7.13   By observing the tidal stream flowing around the Fairway buoy as it is passed.

Chapter 9

9.1   The buoy is an East Cardinal located to the east of a hazard. You should pass to the east of the buoy leaving it to port.

9.2   a) West Cardinal mark.
b) The danger is to the east of the mark.

9.3   **294°T to 304°T**

Chapter 10

10.1   a) This is an International Port Traffic Signal indicating a serious emergency.
b) Stand off and tune to the Port Control channel (usually either channel 12 or 14) on the VHF radio.

Chapter 12

12.1 a)
Tides HW Dartmouth on 26 July is 1204 BST, neap tides. LW is 1743.

Tidal streams Off entrance NE from HW−2 (1004) to HW+4 (1604); SW from LW−2 (1543) to LW+4 (2143).

Entrance waypoint 50° 19'.0N   3° 32'.5W.

Approach From 1M east of Start Point set a course of 030°T (035°M) towards the Entrance Waypoint keeping at least one mile offshore. Look for a conspicuous Day Beacon which is on the hillside just to the east of the entrance. Identify Homestone red buoy to port and then set a course towards Castle Ledge green buoy which should be left to starboard.

Entrance From Castle Ledge buoy set a course of 325°T (330°M) to leave Checkstone red buoy off Castle Point to port. Follow centre of channel until it opens out between the towns of Kingswear and Dartmouth.

Berths The Dartmouth Yacht Club and Dart Marina are on the port hand shore and the Royal Dart Yacht Club and Darthaven Marina in Kingswear to starboard. Look out for *visitors* pontoon or berths.

12.1 (b)

Approach and Entrance Head for the Entrance Waypoint keeping Start Point light (Fl (3) 10s) on a bearing between 215°M and 225°M. Watch out for rough seas off Skerries Bank and for yellow unlit racing buoys in the approaches to the Dart river. Identify Kingswear light (Iso WRG 3s) and approach it in the white sector on a course of 330°T (335°M) leaving Castle Ledge (Fl G 5s) to starboard and Checkstone (Fl (2) R 5s) to port. Identify Dartmouth (Bayards Cove) light (Fl WRG 2s) on port bow and alter course to 290°T (295°M) to stay within the white sector until the harbour opens up to starboard.

12.2 (a)

The lighthouse, near the extremity of Portland Bill, is a white circular tower (43 m high) with a red band. At the point of the Bill is a conspicuous white beacon 18 m high. By night the characteristics of the light are: Fl (4) 20s; but between the bearings of 244°T to 221°T and 117°T to 141°T the four flashes gradually reduce to one flash.

12.2 (b)

Anvil Point light is on a white tower 45 m high. The characteristics of the light are: Fl 10s.

Chapter 14

See Fig A14A for 14.1 to 14.3 and Fig 14B for 14.4 to 14.7.

14.1 a) **50° 12′.5N 3° 38′.0W**
Course 045°T. Water track 050°T.
Tidal stream at HW−1: 066°T 1.0kn.
b) The ground track passes straight through the overfalls.

14.2 **50° 03′.8N 3° 47′.2W**
Course 215°T. Water track 220°T.
Tidal stream at HW−5: 243°T 1.0kn.

14.3 a) **50° 16′.4N 3° 30′.3W**. Yes; the two position lines intersect at right angles.

b) **50° 05′.0N 3° 31′.8W**
Course and water track 195°T.
Tidal stream at HW+1: 059°T 2.0k.
Tidal stream at HW+2: 053°T 1.8kn (for 30 minutes, plot 0.9M).

14.4 **50° 09′.5N 3° 37′.0W**
Course and water track 215°T.
Tidal stream at HW+1: 059°T 2.0kn (for 30 minutes, plot 1.0M).

14.5 **314°C. 1827**
Distance to go 12.0M.
Tidal stream at HW+2: 053° 1.8kn.
Water track 307°T.
Speed made good 10.7kn, time taken 1hr 7 mins.

14.6 **148°C. 0802**
Distance to go 9.6M. Use half hour vector.
Tidal stream at HW−5: 243°T 2.0kn (for 30 minutes, plot 1.0M).
Water track 146°T.
Distance made good 9.0M, speed made good 18.0kn.
Time taken 32 mins.

14.7 The Decca position is wrong.
The correct position is **50° 14′.8N 3° 29′.0W**.

Chapter 19

19.1 A trip line is a light line, one end of which is secured to the crown of the anchor and the other to a small buoy. It should be used when it is suspected that there are obstructions on the seabed which may foul the anchor. It is used to free a foul anchor by pulling it up by its crown.

19.2 **16 metres**

19.3 Sufficient chain or warp for the prevailing conditions should be let out. Suitable transits are selected. An anchor watch may be posted.

MOTORMASTER

19.4
1 Present and expected wind strength and direction.
2 Tidal stream effects.
3 Topography of the coast line.
4 Easy access; important if it is necessary to make a night departure.
5 Good holding ground free from obstructions.
6 Clear of hazards and other boats at all states of the tide when swinging.
7 Sufficient depth of water for the duration of the stay.
8 Where the boat has sufficient anchor cable at all states of the tide.
9 Clear of channels frequently used by other boats.
10 If going ashore, near a landing site.
11 Away from moored boats and small craft moorings.

19.5 To stop the boat yawing in strong winds, there should be an angle of about 40° between the two anchors both led from the bows. To limit the swinging circle in a tidal stream, both anchors are lead from the bows; the heaviest one into the strongest tidal stream.

Chapter 21

21.1 The Shipping Forecast, Navtex and Weatherfax and Metfax Marine.

21.2 Niton Coast Radio Station weather bulletin 0733 GMT. Inshore Waters Forecast on BBC Radio 4 at 0550.

21.3 A cold front has passed over Poole. The southwesterly wind will have established a wave pattern from the southwest. When the wind changes to northwest, a new northwesterly wave pattern is created which is initially superimposed on the previous pattern. For some hours, therefore, there can be very confused seas. There are tidal eddies off Anvil Point and many overfalls off St Albans Head. It would be better to delay the passage until the wind decreases and the sea settles down.

21.4
a) Less than **2 miles**
b) **35 to 45 knots**
c) **Force 7**
d) **Force 4**
e) **12 to 24 hours**

21.5
a) A cold front
b) see Fig A21A
c) The report from coastal station Channel Light Vessel shows that a cold front is approaching sea area Wight. Northwest gale force 8 is reported at Channel Light Vessel. The forecast for Wight is initially southwest 5 but becoming northwest 6 to 8. For a passage from Cherbourg to Southampton in such conditions, a boat would experience head winds and a rough dangerous sea. Even wind force 5 would be too lively for a small motorboat. The passage should be delayed until the wind decreases and the weather becomes more settled.

21.6
a) Anchorages **C**, **A**, **B**. **A** and **C** are sheltered from the southwest though, with a veering wind, **A** could become steadily more exposed. **B** is open to the south.
b) Anchorages **B**, **C**, **A**. Both **A** and **C** are fairly open to prospective gale force winds. Once the wind has veered to the west, **B** offers long term protection for riding out a gale. **A** would become untenable.

Chapter 22

22.1
a) When there is a danger of the boat sinking or when in the tender.
b) In rough weather especially at night when the crew need to be on the foredeck or if using an outside steering position.

MOTORMASTER

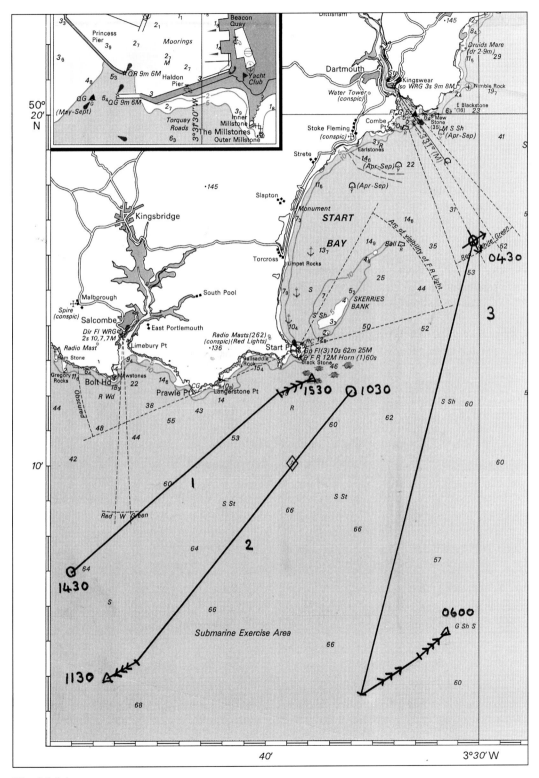

Fig A14A

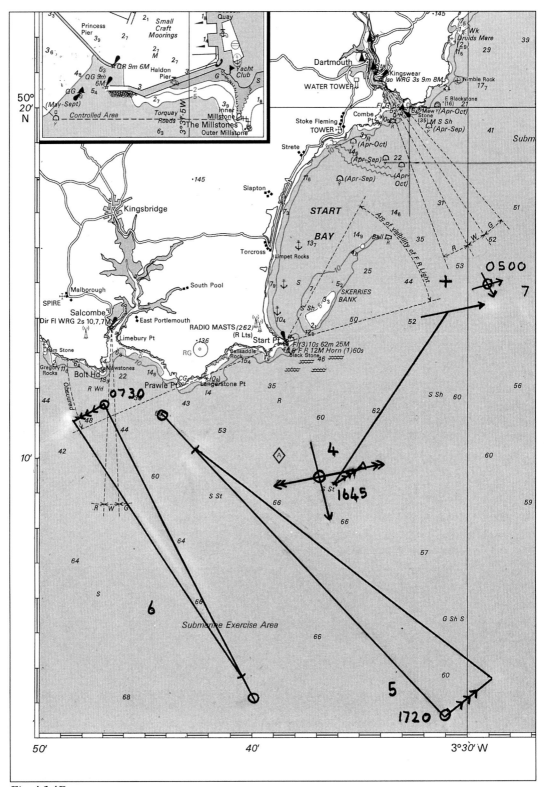

MOTORMASTER

Fig A14B

22.2   a) CO_2 or powder
      b) Powder, foam or CO_2

22.3   1 Stop the engine.
      2 Extinguish all flames.
      3 Turn off fuel and gas at source.
      4 Ventilate the boat.
      5 Find the leak.
      6 Do not use the engine, cooker, heater or naked flame until the leak has been stopped and the boat ventilated.

22.4   a) Two red handflares, two orange handsmokes, two red parachute rockets.
      b) Four red handflares, four red parachute rockets, two orange lifesmokes.

22.5   Immediately before boarding as it could turn over or become damaged if towed.

Chapter 23

23.1
Rule 6
Visibility and volume of traffic, boats stopping ability and manoeuvrability.

23.2
Rule 7
By taking a series of compass bearings of the approaching vessel. If the bearing does not appreciably change then a risk of collision is deemed to exist. Sometimes a risk of collision can exist even when an appreciable bearing change is evident, particularly when approaching a very large vessel, a tug with tow, or a vessel at close range.

23.3
Rules 34 and 35
i   Any of the following: vessel not under command; vessel restricted in her ability to manoeuvre; vessel constrained by her draught; sailing vessel; vessel engaged in fishing; vessel towing or pushing. (Restricted visibility)
ii   I am unsure of your intentions. (Manoeuvring)
iii   I am altering course to starboard. (Manoeuvring)
iv   Power driven vessel making way. (Restricted visibility)
v   My engines are going astern. (Manoeuvring)
vi   I am intending to overtake you on your starboard side. (Manoeuvring)

23.4
Rule 14 A and B both alter course to starboard.
Rule 18 Power vessel A gives way to sailing vessel B.
Rule 15 A gives way to B. She should pass astern of B.
Rule 13 A gives way to B. An overtaking vessel must keep well clear of the overtaken vessel until she is finally passed and clear.

	Before cold front	Passage of cold front	After cold front
Wind strength	5	6–8	8 decreasing to 5
Wind direction	southwest	northwest	northwest
Barometric trend	steady	rising rapidly	rising more slowly
Visibility	poor	poor in showers becoming good	good
Precipitation	rain	heavy showers	occasional showers
Cloud	stratus	cumulus or cumulonimbus	occasional cumulus

Fig A21A

Rule 18 B gives way to A. B should pass astern of A.

Rule 18 A gives way to B. B is restricted in her ability to manoeuvre.

23.5

Rule 27 A vessel restricted in her ability to manoeuvre, underway, stern aspect, probably a dredger.

Rule 23 A power driven vessel less than 50 m in length, underway, starboard aspect.

Rule 28 A vessel constrained by her draught (maybe over 50 m in length), underway, port aspect.

Rule 26 A vessel less than 50 m in length engaged in fishing by trawling, underway, starboard aspect.

Rule 25 Sailing vessel, underway, port aspect.

Rule 30 A vessel at anchor (maybe over 50 m in length), port aspect, not underway.

23.6

Rule 8 Action to avoid collision should be positive, made in good time and clearly apparent to the other vessel.

23.7

Rule 10 With the heading as nearly as practicable to right angles to the general direction of the traffic flow.

23.8

Rule 5 At all times by sight, hearing and all available means.

23.9   Annex IV. Any of the following:
1 Continuous sounding of the fog signalling apparatus.
2 SOS by any method.
3 Radio telephony call MAYDAY.
4 International code flags N over C.
5 A square flag above or below a ball.
6 Red rocket parachute flare or red handflare.
7 An orange smoke signal.
8 Slowly and repeatedly raising and lowering the outstretched arms.

Chapter 24

24.1 The crew member is most likely suffering from hypothermia and every effort should be made to stop further heat loss. The following actions should be taken:
1 Remove to a sheltered place and take off wet clothes.
2 Cover with blankets or sleeping bag and wrap in a plastic bag.
3 Place in a horizontal position. Body warmth can be transferred from another person in the sleeping bag.
4 Keep in a warm place such as near the engine.
5 If conscious and there are no injuries give hot sweet drinks and chocolate.
6 If unconscious place in the recovery position and watch in case vomiting occurs, breathing ceases, or the heart stops.
7 If any of the above happen, take the appropriate action.
8 Any casualty who has had water in his lungs should be referred to hospital as soon as possible.

24.2
1 Apply pressure to the wound using a sterile pad.
2 Secure the pad.
3 If the wound bleeds through the pad, apply a further dressing over the top.
4 Elevate the limb.
5 If bleeding does not stop, apply pressure to the brachial artery using the fingers, but for not more than 15 minutes.
6 Treat for shock.
7 Refer to a doctor as soon as possible.

24.3 a) Immediately cool the affected area by immersion in cold water. This should be done for at least 10 minutes.
b) 1 Remove anything likely to reduce circulation such as a wrist watch. The burned area may swell up.
2 Cut away loose clothing but leave any adhering to the burn.

MOTORMASTER

3 Cover with non–fluffy dressing; clingfilm is excellent.

4 Treat for shock.

5 If severe seek medical assistance.

24.4

1 Place in a cool place out of the sun.

2 Sponge with cold water and apply calamine lotion.

3 Treat for heatstroke if necessary.

4 If severely burned refer to a doctor.

24.5

1 Lay the casualty down and immobilise the leg with a splint.

2 Check the extremities of the limb to see that they are not blue as the splint may be too tight.

3 Elevate the limb.

4 Treat for shock.

5 Refer to hospital as soon as possible for X–ray.

MOTORMASTER

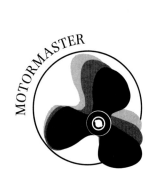

GLOSSARY

abaft Aft of any particular point on the vessel.

abeam At right angles to the line of the keel.

aft Towards the stern or rear of the vessel.

air mass A mass of air which is largely similar in a horizontal direction.

amidships Midway between stem and stern.

anabatic wind A warm wind that flows up slopes during the day in sunny conditions.

anenometer An instrument for measuring wind speed.

anti-cyclone A region of high barometric pressure.

athwart From side to side.

avast To stop, to hold fast.

aweigh Term to indicate that the anchor has broken out of the ground.

a-bracket Fitting supporting the propeller shaft.

back An anti-clockwise shift of the wind.

ballast Iron or lead placed in the bottom of a ship to improve her stability.

bar A shoal in the entrance to a harbour.

beacon An aid to navigation set on the shore or on rocks.

beam Extreme width of a vessel. The direction when abeam; at right angles to the fore-and-aft line.

bear away To steer a boat away from the direction of the wind.

bearing The direction of an object expressed in compass notation, eg 180°C.

Beaufort scale A measurement of wind strength.

belay To make a rope fast.

bend A type of knot.

bight Any part of a rope between its ends. A curve, or cove, on a coastline.

bilge The curve of the underwater part of the vessel nearest the keel.

binnacle The box which holds the steering compass.

bitter end The last part of a rope or cable secured on board.

bluff Steep shore.

bollard Post on a quay or deck for securing a ship's mooring lines.

boot-topping A narrow painted band on the waterline.

bow Forward part of a vessel.

bower anchor The main anchor carried in the bows.

breast line Ropes forward and aft secured to the jetty at right angles to the boat.

bring up To stop.

broach to To turn accidentally broadside to the wind and sea.

bulkheads Partitions fore-and-aft or athwartships forming separate compartments.

bulwarks A vessel's topsides that extend above the deck.

buoy A float which may have a distinguishing name, shape, colour or light.

burgee Pennant (pointed) shaped flag with a design indicating the yacht club to which the owner belongs.

cable One tenth of a nautical mile. Anchor chain.

capstan A vertical cylindrical device for veering out or hoisting the anchor chain.

cardinal mark Indicating navigable water on the named side, ie north, south, east or west, of the mark.

carry way To continue to move through the water.

carvel Edge to edge planking for a vessel's hull.

cast off To let go.

cavitation Vibration and loss of power caused by tiny air bubbles bursting against the propeller and causing pitting on the blades.

chart datum The level to which drying heights and soundings on a chart are related.

check To stop slowly a vessel's movement. To ease out a rope slowly.

chine The fore-and-aft line of the hull where the bilge turns upwards towards the topsides of the hull.

cleat A two-pronged device for making ropes fast.

clinker Planking where one edge overlaps the lower plank.

coachroof A raised structure to improve headroom below deck.

cold front The boundary between the advancing cold air at the rear of a depression and the warm sector.

companion Ladder in a boat.

compass swing Procedure for finding the deviation (error) of a compass.

con To give orders to the helmsman.

counter The overhanging portion of the stern.

course The direction a vessel steers.

course to steer The course relating to the compass used by the helmsman.

cradle A framework to support a vessel out of the water.

crown The point where the arms of an anchor meet the shank.

crutch Metal fitting that drops into the gunwale of a boat to take an oar.

cyclone A name given to tropical revolving storms in the Bay of Bengal and the Arabian Sea.

cyclonic Refers to wind circulating anti-clockwise round a low pressure area in northern latitudes.

davit A crane for hoisting, lowering and holding boats in a vessel.

dead reckoning The position found from course steered and distance run.

deadweight Total weight of a vessel: its displacement.

deck log The record of events on a ship, especially navigational.

deckhead Underside of the deck. The roof of a cabin.

deep Deepwater channel between shoals.

depression A region characterised by low barometric pressure.

depth contour A line on a chart joining points of equal depth.

deviation Compass error caused by magnetism of the vessel.

dew Water droplets formed by condensation of water vapour from the air.

dew point The lowest temperature to which air can be cooled without causing condensation.

dip To lower and raise the ensign in salute.

dog watches The two-hour watches from 1600–1800 and 1800–2000.

dolphin A pile structure for mooring in a harbour.

dowse To extinguish a light. To spray with water.

draught The depth of water occupied by a vessel.

drift The distance covered in a given time due to the movement of the current or tidal stream.

drogue A sea anchor: a cone shaped canvas bag to which a vessel lies in heavy weather to keep her bows pointing into the waves.

ebb The period during which the tide is falling or flowing away from the land.

echo sounder An electronic instrument to measure the depth of water.

eddy Circular motion of water unconnected with general water movement.

ensign The flag flown at the stern that denotes a vessel's nationality.

estimated position The best approximation of a boat's position allowing for leeway, set and drift.

fairlead a fitting for leading a rope over an obstruction.

fairway A channel used for shipping, normally the centre of an approach channel.

fathom Nautical measurement of a depth of 6ft (1.8m).

fend off To push off.

fender Rubber, plastic or rope pad to prevent chafe between vessels or between a vessel and the quayside.

fetch The distance that the wind has covered from the weather shore to the boat.

MOTORMASTER

fiddle A lip frame around horizontal surfaces to stop objects sliding off.

fix A position obtained by taking accurate bearings.

flare A marine pyrotechnic used as a distress signal. The overhang of a vessel's bow.

flashing Navigation light where the duration of the light is less than the dark period.

flood The rising tide.

fore and aft The centre line of the vessel in line with the keel.

forward Towards the bow.

foul Opposite to clear:'foul berth', 'foul anchor', 'foul bottom'. A contrary tidal stream.

frap To bind ropes together to prevent flapping.

freeboard The distance from the waterline to the edge of the deck.

freshen An increasing wind.

front The line of separation on the earth's surface between cold and warm air masses.

gale Wind of force 8 or 9 on the Beaufort scale (34 to 47 knots).

galley The kitchen of a boat.

gimbals A pivoted frame to allow a compass or stove to remain horizontal.

ground, to A ship grounds when the keel touches the seabed.

ground track The path of a boat over the ground.

gunwale The top rail of a boat.

gust A rapid fluctuation in the strength of the wind.

guy A rope used to control a spar or derrick.

handsomely Gently or slowly.

hard A slope of hard material used for beaching small vessels.

hawse pipes Pipes leading down through the bows through which are led the anchor chains.

hawser A heavy rope used for mooring, kedging, warping, towing or as a temporary anchor cable.

head sea Waves and wind from ahead.

heading The direction in which the boat is pointing.

heads The toilets on a boat.

heaving line A light line, knotted at one end, to throw ashore as a messenger for a mooring line.

heel To lean over from upright.

helm The tiller or wheel.

hitch A knot used to make a rope fast to a spar.

holding ground The type of bottom (seabed) for an anchor.

holiday An unpainted spot in a vessel.

house flag The rectangular personal flag of the boat's owner.

hull The structure of a vessel below deck level.

hurricane A name given to a tropical revolving storm in the West Indies.

inshore Towards the shore.

inversion When air temperature increases with altitude.

isobars Lines drawn between points of equal barometric pressure, on a weather chart.

isophase Navigation light where the duration of light and dark are equal.

jack staff Small staff in the bows from which a flag may be flown.

jury rig A makeshift rig to get a vessel to safety.

katabatic wind A cool wind that flows down slopes, usually at night.

kedge A lightweight anchor.

keel The heavy backbone of a vessel running fore-and-aft. The bottom of a vessel.

king spoke The spoke of the steering wheel which is upright when the helm is amidships.

knot One nautical mile per hour.

landfall First sight of the land from seaward.

lashing Securing with a rope.

lateral mark navigation mark on the port and starboard sides of a well-defined channel.

launch To slide a vessel into the water. A small motor tender.

lazy An extra rope; a lazy painter.

lead The lead weight at the end of a lead line used to find the depth of water.

leading marks Marks or lights that are brought into line to indicate the channel or best approach.

lee side The side away from the wind direction.

leeshore Shore on to which the wind is blowing.

leeward Towards the sheltered side.

leeway The sideways drift of a vessel caused by the wind.

lifeline Lines stretched fore-and-aft for the crew to hold on.

line squall A violent squall usually associated with the passage of a cold front.

list To heel over.

log An instrument for recording the distance run.

log book The record of events on a ship, especially navigational.

loom The reflection of light on the clouds when a light is below the horizon. The handle of an oar.

lubber line The line on the inside of a compass bowl indicating the fore and aft line of the boat.

make To attain.

make fast To secure.

make water To leak.

marry Bring two ropes together.

meridian A north–south line running through any point.

messenger A light line tied to a hawser or warp to pass round a winch where the hawser is too heavy to handle.

midships To centralise the rudder.

moor To moor is to lie with two anchors down. A vessel is moored to a jetty when made fast with several mooring lines.

neap tides When the rise and fall of tide is least; when the moon is in quadrature.

neaped A ship aground when there is insufficient rise of tide to float her.

nothing to port Do not steer any further to port.

nothing to starboard Do not steer any further to starboard.

occlusion When a cold front is overtaking a warm front and has lifted the warm sector from the earth's surface.

occulting Navigation light with a duration of light period more than the dark.

offing To seaward.

painter The rope secured to the bow of a dinghy or tender by which it is towed.

pay out To ease out a rope.

pitching A ship's movement in a seaway in a fore-and-aft direction.

polar front The front between the polar maritime and tropical maritime air masses.

pooped A heavy sea has entered the boat over the stern.

port The left-hand side of the boat looking forward.

quarter Midway between beam and dead astern.

race A local area of disturbed water.

racon Beacon giving a characteristic response when triggered by the ship's radar.

radiobeacon A radio transmitter from which the navigator can obtain a position line.

range a cable To flake down, ie lay in a figure of eight pattern, lengths of cable on deck.

range of tide The difference in height between successive high and low waters.

reef A ridge of rocks.

rhumb line A course that crosses all meridians at the same angle.

ridge An extension of an area of high barometric pressure.

riding light An anchor light.

round turn A complete turn around a bollard to keep the strain on a rope under tension.

samson post A strong post in the fore part of a vessel to secure a towline or anchor cable.

scud Fragments of cloud drifting rapidly in a strong wind.

scuppers Holes in bulwarks to allow water to drain from deck.

scuttles Round holes in a ship's side for ventilation and light.

sea breeze Onshore wind caused by warming of the land on a sunny day.

MOTORMASTER

seacock A valve in a pipe connected to the sea.

set The direction towards which a current or tidal stream is flowing.

sheer The rise of a ship's deck towards the bow or stern from amidships.

ship To take on board.

skeg A fixed vertical fin to which the rudder is attached.

slack water Stationary tidal stream.

slip Slope for launching boats.

sole The floor of the cockpit or cabin.

sound/sounding To measure the depth of water.

spring A mooring rope to prevent a vessel moving fore-and-aft when secured alongside a quay.

spring tides The greatest range of tides; when the moon is full or new.

squall A strong wind that increases suddenly, lasts for a few minutes, then rapidly decreases.

stanchion Vertical support for lifelines running around edge of deck.

stand off Head away from the shore or some obstacle.

stand on Maintain course.

starboard The right-hand side of a ship facing forward.

steady Order to the helmsman to maintain the course being steered.

steerage way When a vessel is moving fast enough to respond to her helm.

stem The forward continuation of the keel to deck level.

stern The aft continuation of the keel to deck level.

surge To allow a rope under tension to slip on a capstan or bollard.

synoptic chart The weather conditions over a given area at a given instant of time.

tackle A combination of ropes and blocks.

taff-rail A rail around the stern of a vessel.

thwarts Planks placed across a boat to form seats.

tidal stream The horizontal movement of the sea caused by the tide.

tide The periodic rise and fall in the level of the sea.

tiller Lever for turning the rudder.

track The path between one position and another.

transducer A sensor.

transit A line formed when two distant objects are in line one behind the other.

transom The flat stern of a boat.

trick A period at the helm.

trough An extension of an area of low barometric pressure.

tumble home Where a ship's sides are inclined inwards above the water line.

turning short round Turning a vessel within as small a circle as possible.

typhoon A name given to tropical revolving storms in the China Sea and the northwest Pacific Ocean.

under way When a vessel is not made fast to the ground.

up and down When an anchor cable is vertical; the anchor is just lifting off the seabed.

veer A clockwise shift of the wind.

veer out To ease out a cable.

wake Disturbed water astern of a vessel as it moves ahead.

warm front The boundary between the warm air sector and the cold air that precedes it.

warp Rope used for mooring.

warping Moving a vessel by means of ropes and hawsers.

wash The waves caused by a vessel's progress through the water.

watches Periods of duty for members of the crew.

water track The path of a boat through the water.

weather helm A boat has weather helm when she has a tendency to turn towards the wind.

weather side The side upon which the wind is blowing.

weigh To lift the anchor off the ground.

wind rode Where an anchored vessel is lying to the wind rather than the tide.

yaw When the ship's head is swung by the action of the waves.

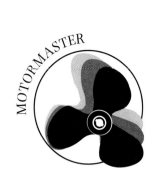

INDEX

Admiralty Notices to
  Mariners 26
air masses 149-54
almanacs 93
anabatic wind 142
anchors 126-31
  chain and warp 130-2
  choosing 134
  fouled 135, 136
  sizes 130
  stowage 132
  trip line 135

back bearings 75
Beaufort Wind Scale 166,
  167
bleeding 200
boat speed 96
bora 143
bowline (knot) 124, 131
breezes, land and sea 141-2
Bruce anchor 128
buoyage 62-5
buoy, picking up 139-40
burns and scalds 201

canals 86
cardinal marks 65
Chart 50011 Symbols and
  Abbreviations 25
chart measurement scales
  22
chart plotters, electronic
  112
chart display and
  information system
  (ECDIS) 112
charts 21-35
  cautions 26
  corrections 26
  publishers 26
  scale 23
  symbols 24
clearing bearings 74-6
clove hitch (knot) 124
coastal passage plan 215-
  16
chart abbreviations 16
chart datum 38
charts, electronic 105
chartwork 94-104
chest injury 201
choking 204
cleating a rope 124
Coastal Skipper RYA course
  v, vi

Coastguard 90-1
collision avoidance 115
collision rules 187-96
compasses
  adjustment 17
  card type 13
  deviation 17
  electronic 14, 18-19
  error 15
  hand bearing compass
    14, 19
  monocular fluxgate
    compass 15
  variation 15, 16
compass rose 16, 25
concussion 206
coral graze 204
course to steer 94-5
CQR anchor 129
cross waves 144
crossing situation 192
Customs and Excise 233
cuts 204

Danforth anchor 129, 133
Day Skipper RYA course v,
  vi
dead reckoning position 99,
  100, 102
Decca Navigator 107-8
depression (weather) 150-3
depth contours 25, 99
depths of water, calculating
  51
deviation, compass 17
dipping lights 70-1
direction, finding 32
dislocations and fractures
  204
distance, measuring 32, 34
distress calls 117-19
distress signals 196
dressing ship 122

electronic compasses 18-19
electronic navigation
  systems 105-15
electronic position
  indicating
  system, setting up 114
emergency position
  indicating radio
  beacons (EPIRB) 120
engine control 6-12
engine performance data
  11

engines
  control 6-12
  diesel 6
  four-stroke petrol 6
  fuel consumption 7
  two-stroke petrol 6
ensigns and burgees 121
error, compass 15
estimated position 100,
  101, 102
etesian (wind) 143
eye injuries 206

facsimile receivers 120
fetch 142
figure of eight knot 124
fire extinguishers 176-7
fire prevention 178-9
first aid 199-211
  kit 205
Fisherman anchor 127
fisherman's bend (knot)
  124, 131
fish hook injury 204
fixes 98
fixing position 98
flags 121-2
flares 182-4
fluxgate compass 14, 19
fog 145-7
fog signals 93, 194-5
forecasting, weather 155-
  68
fuel consumption 7-12
fuel management 6-12
fuel tanks 12

Global Maritime Distress
  and Safety System
  (GMDSS) 120
global positioning system
  (GPS) 108-10
grapnel anchor 128
gregale 143
ground track 95

Harbour, approaches to
  58-9, 81
harbour authorities 92
harbour entry 60-1
headlands, identifying 82-3
headwounds 206
heart attacks 207
heat exhaustion 208
heat stroke 208
helicopter rescue 180, 181

HF radio telephone 119
high pressure systems 149
hull types 1-2
hyperbolic navigation
  systems 106-7
hypothermia 208

Inmarsat 120
insect stings 209
integrated navigation
  systems 111-13
internal bleeding 209
International Certificate of
  Competence (ICC) vi
international code flags
  122
International Maritime
  Organisation (IMO) 92
International Regulations
  for Preventing
  Collisions at Sea
  (IRPCS) 187-96
isolated danger marks 65

jellyfish stings 209

katabatic wind 142
kedge anchor 128
khamsin 143
knots 124-25

IALA buoyage system 62
lateral marks 64
latitude 21-22, 29
leading marks and lights 69
levanter 143
levache 142
liferafts 174-5
lighthouses 66-71
lights 66-72, 194-5
light signals 93
locks 86-7
longitude 21-22, 29
Loran C 108
low pressure systems 147-8

man overboard 180-2
marks for fixes 98
marks, types of 64-5
Mayday calls 117-18
medical advice by radio
  119
Mediterranean mooring
  140
Mediterranean winds
  142-3